Managing Menopause Naturally

Before, During, and Forever

Emily Kane, N.D., L.Ac.

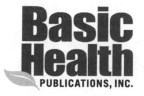
Basic Health
PUBLICATIONS, INC.

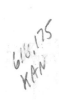

The information contained in this book is based upon the research and personal and professional experiences of the author. It is not intended as a substitute for consulting with your physician or other healthcare provider. Any attempt to diagnose and treat an illness should be done under the direction of a healthcare professional.

The publisher does not advocate the use of any particular healthcare protocol but believes the information in this book should be available to the public. The publisher and author are not responsible for any adverse effects or consequences resulting from the use of the suggestions, preparations, or procedures discussed in this book. Should the reader have any questions concerning the appropriateness of any procedures or preparation mentioned, the author and the publisher strongly suggest consulting a professional healthcare advisor.

Basic Health Publications, Inc.

8200 Boulevard East

North Bergen, NJ 07047

1-201-868-8336

Library of Congress Cataloging-in-Publication Data

Kane, Emily.
    Managing menopause naturally : before, during, and forever / Emily Kane.
       p. cm.
    ISBN 1-59120-063-6
    1. Menopause—Popular works. 2. Middle-aged women—Health and
hygiene. I. Title.
    RG186.K3625   2004
    618.1'75—dc22

                                                        2003023142

Editor: Roberta W. Waddell
Typesetting/Book design: Gary A. Rosenberg
Cover design: Mike Stromberg

Printed in the United States of America

10   9   8   7   6   5   4   3   2   1

Contents

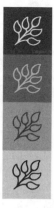

Acknowledgments

Heartfelt thanks to my family, Bret Schmiege and Katherine Kane, who actually left me alone in the house on Tuesday afternoons for several months to let me write this book. I love you, and thank you for loving me. I also wish to express my great fondness and respect for my parents, Ed and Phyllis Kane, who have always encouraged me to pursue my own interests. And I place my hands in namaste and bow to my many teachers at Bastyr University; an incomplete list includes Cathy Rogers, Bruce Milliman, Elias Illya, Jon Hibbs, Jane Guiltinan, Rich Frederickson, Maureen O'Keefe, Molly Linton, Silena Heron, and Jeff Basom. I also deeply appreciate what I have learned about women's bodies from Drs. Lili Tang, Tori Hudson, and Christianne Northrup. Many thanks to my editor, Bobby Waddell, for organizing the text to make it a more useful book. Bobby's pragmatic, no-nonsense approach to editing was very detail-oriented, but never lost sight of the big picture. Mostly, I thank the community of Juneau, Alaska, especially the downtown gang centering around Rainbow Foods (Dave Ottoson and Linda Cohen) for helping me to grow as a physician. Blessings to you all. Blessings to us all.

Introduction

This book is designed to help women manage menopause naturally, beginning with the transition from regular monthly menstruation and its accompanying possibility of pregnancy to a new freedom called menopause. By the year 2015, 50 percent of the women in the United States will be menopausal, and three-quarters of these women will have symptoms. Contrary to the current interests and practices of our medical establishment, however, menopause is *not* a disease, and it does not usually require pharmaceutical medication. (Pregnancy and childbirth aren't diseases either, for that matter.) Women are supposed to stop menstruating at a certain age. When and how we originally go from girl to woman and have our first period (menarche) is determined by many factors (hormonal, dietary, emotional, and environmental), and there are just as many factors that contribute to menopause at the cessation of menstruation and the end of our fertile years. Menopause is a gift that allows us to live many more years without periods, without the specter of an unwanted pregnancy, and without the potential roller coaster of premenstrual moodiness. It technically begins twelve months to the day after the last menstrual period, and may be rocky at times, but this book is intended as a road map to help you navigate through it smoothly and emerge radiantly healthy.

Part One has ten chapters detailing the top ten complaints of hormonal shifting, including breast tenderness, bone loss, and hot flashes. Chapter 1 explains which hormones are involved in menstruation and their role in menopause. Each chapter in Part One has a final summary for quick reference. Part Two introduces and explains some of the exceptional tools and techniques you can use to create a natural, wholesome transition to menopause. Part Three describes the major hormonal control systems of the body—the adrenals, ovaries, and thyroid gland—so you will understand what is *really going on* in your body during this transition. Part Four is an overview of how to stay healthy and happy beyond menopause, with chapters on maintaining a functional immune system, preventing heart disease, and the connection between cancer and diet.

My bias as a naturopathic doctor is to work with what nature offers: fresh air, pure water, organic food, and most of all, the incredible blend of what makes up a person. The physical machine, the realm of feelings and emotions, and the complexity of the intellect are all equally important players in our health and well-being. My perspective, and my goal for the patients under my care, is not merely to be rid of illness, but to achieve optimum health and well-being. Remember, hormonal transition is *normal*. You are not sick, and you probably don't need drugs or to go to the hospital.

It is tricky to get an unbiased opinion about medical approaches to menopause when the information is coming from doctors, and even more so from pharmaceutical company representatives, who have a financial interest in your dependence upon their products and services. The purpose of this book is to open your mind to the possibility of natural self-care as you go through menopause or any other life transition. Ultimately, a commitment to healthy choices in diet, relationships, and daily activities is what creates a permanent and solid foundation for well-being.

I would like to briefly address a few menopause myths.

✗ **In the old days, women didn't live much beyond menopause, but modern women live much longer so their estrogen must be replaced.** One hundred years ago, women *did* die sooner, but these deaths were mostly related to childbirth. Either the infant girl died, or the young mother giving birth died because of blood loss or infection. Even hundreds of years ago, women who survived infancy and childbirth often lived to old age. Further, women continue to secrete estrogen from their adrenal glands and fat cells their entire lives. Menopausal and perimenopausal women have a naturally appropriate amount of estrogen production for these phases of their lives.

✗ **Menopause causes arthritis, heart disease, osteoporosis, and all sorts of other chronic diseases.** Actually, unhealthy *aging* causes these problems. Men typically acquire heart disease earlier than women and they are not exempt from osteoporosis (bone loss). I sincerely hope this book will help you gain a great deal of practical information about healthy aging.

✗ **Menopause turns women into raging terrors** (I'm avoiding the "B" word here). Actually, younger women are more likely to fly into rages and get moody, for two reasons. First, they have a lot more hormonal activity than a menopausal woman. And second, just like good wine, women tend to mellow with age.

✗ **Menopause should be treated with standard hormones.** This is what the drug companies would like you to believe. The truth is, there is no one-size-fits-all solution to hormone replacement, even assuming it is needed at all. Standard prescription hormones have been proven to be harmful. Luckily, there are safer alternatives available in plant based and bioidentical hormones, which are explained in Chapter 11, the opening chapter of Part Two.

The primary message of this book is that menopause is a transition—it is *not* an illness. The transition may be long and gradual or it may be abrupt. Each woman is unique and will experience her passage differently. A number of general concepts that hold true are presented in these pages. A highly important one is to stay committed to excellent health and focused on cultivating a deep sense of joy. We're only sure we've got this life—we might as well make it stellar!

PART ONE

Symptoms of Hormonal Change

1.

Weird Periods— Or Maybe They Were Never Regular

The orchestration of menstruation is as complex as any symphony. Our monthly periods are a result of hormonal changes, glandular secretions, and a system of temporary arteries within the uterine lining. For convenience, the first day of bleeding is considered to be day one of the menstrual cycle, which is generally twenty-nine days in length. The first half of the menstrual cycle is called the follicular phase, because follicles, which protect the clusters of maturing eggs within the ovaries, begin to ripen. This follicular development is responding to a brain secretion called FSH (follicular stimulating hormone) and is initially independent of other hormonal influence. Levels of the hormone estrogen are relatively low at this point, but the rising levels of FSH stimulate both the FSH and LH (luteinizing hormone) receptors in the follicles. The activated FSH and LH receptors, in turn, stimulate production of estrogen hormone in the follicles. LH is the hormone that provokes ovulation (the release of egg(s) from the ovary).

What Estrogen Does

The secretion of estrogen in the follicles causes a gradual increase in the production of cervical mucus that peaks when the monthly estrogen secretion reaches its maximum level at ovulation. Nature has done this to allow ovulation to coincide with a moist, slippery vagina, a lowered uterus, and a ferning pattern in the cervical mucus, all provided by the surge in estrogen levels. The beautiful fernlike pattern in the cervical mucus looks like an evergreen forest seen from a distance, or like cracks on a large sheet of thin ice. The purpose of this ferning pattern, besides entertaining biologists and medical students, is to provide tracks to guide the sperm up toward the open end of the uterus, called the os. Meanwhile, the egg in the ovary is almost ready to drop. (The follicle producing the most estrogen will ripen into a mature egg.) Eventually, around day fifteen in the monthly cycle, the increased estrogen levels trigger a surge of LH, which, along with increased enzymatic activity around the chosen follicle, causes ovulation, which is the release of the mature egg. Ovulation stimulates progesterone production, which comes in very handy in the event of a successful conception.

What Progesterone Does

The second half of the menstrual cycle is called the luteal phase. When the egg is released from the follicle, it bursts through the ovary wall in order to reach the uterus via the fallopian tubes. The ovarian follicle emerges from a mass of yellow cells called the *corpus luteum* (Latin for "yellow body"). The *corpus luteum* then begins to produce progesterone, which supports the growth of an embryo.

Maybe a viable sperm is already lurking in the womb, maybe not. After the LH surge, progesterone begins to wane unless the implantation of an embryo occurs. If pregnancy does occur, hCG (human chorionic gonadatropin) begins to be secreted by the placenta, maintaining the *corpus luteum* for continued progesterone production until the placenta takes over. It is the hCG levels that are tested in home pregnancy kits; during the first weeks of pregnancy, hCG doubles weekly.

Why Do We Bleed?

If pregnancy does not occur, the corpus luteum dies within twelve days, resulting in rapidly declining levels of progesterone. At the end of the monthly cycles, the endometrium contains newly suffused, coiled arteries that have been building in preparation for ovulation and pregnancy. These now constrict, cutting off oxygen to themselves and the uterine lining, leading to tissue deterioration. At this point the endometrial lining of the uterus begins to slough off. Blood from the ruptured, coiled arteries and disrupted endometrial cells comprises the menstrual flow. Large clots in the menses are chunks of tissue that don't have time to undergo liquefaction before they are pushed into the vagina, and they are indicative of heavy bleeding. The average blood loss during a period is about one-quarter of a cup, and the average duration of a menstrual period is five days: two days of heavier bleeding, then three days tapering off.

Running Out of Eggs

As Chapter 18 on the ovaries describes, women lose their eggs rapidly, even before their own birth. Today's woman is likely to live thirty years beyond her so-called fertile years. Because women have fewer pregnancies today, the average woman will have more ovulations and more periods earlier in her life, and will lose her eggs faster than a woman living 100 years ago or more. Running out of eggs sooner means fewer ovulations later, and fewer ovulations means less progesterone will be produced. This is the cornerstone of understanding what leads up to menopause. Progesterone goes away first, followed by the decline of various estrogens, and finally, the tapering off of the testosterone. However, it is important to realize that although progesterone is no longer produced after the cessation of ovulation, women still continue to produce considerable amounts of estrogen and testosterone from their fat cells and their adrenal glands after menopause. The many symptoms that can ensue from diminishing hormone levels will be discussed one by one in the following chapters.

When Do We Stop Bleeding?

First, let's talk about the weird periods that can start to happen years before hormonal changes are detectable by blood or saliva tests. These weird periods are simply the changing pattern of your menstrual cycle and often the very first hint that menopause is coming, even though it may not be coming for years—maybe as many as ten years. Women can and do get pregnant well into these perimenopausal years, weird periods and all. (I can personally attest to that, having birthed my first child at age forty-two after several months of less-than-regular menstrual periods.)

Sometimes, if you're lucky with your genes, your periods might get lighter and lighter, and further and further apart, and then quietly go away forever. Most women are not so lucky, even with good genes. A typical age to stop bleeding is fifty-one, but a few women continue their menstrual cycles well into their sixties. Many women begin premenopause (also called perimenopause) about four years before that, on average at age forty-seven. Knowing when your mother began her hormonal changes can be useful for you because daughters will often follow their mothers' patterns (although many women of my mother's generation experienced surgical menopause, which is much less likely to be used today to treat the symptoms of hormonal change). The average menstrual cycle lasts approximately one month, which is why women who have regular bleeding can time their periods to lunar cycles. A variety of factors can cause this to vary, including travel (especially west to east travel across time zones), stress, dietary changes, and exposure to unusual odors or different levels of light. It is quite normal to have irregularly timed periods as we approach menopause. Most women will experience this to some degree, and will also find that it is more common for the cycles to get shorter than for the periods to get further apart.

What If My Bleeding Is Actually Getting Heavier?

Because of waning progesterone in the perimenopausal phase leading up to menopause, the endometrium tends to shed early. Additionally, a relatively higher concentration of estrogen may exist, also because of lower progesterone. Estrogen is the hormone responsible for the thickening of the uterine lining, a process also known as endometrial proliferation. The net result of this lowering of progesterone in combination with a higher concentration of estrogen is shorter cycles with heavier periods. Not fun. In cases of extremely heavy bleeding (a cup or more of blood per cycle), other more serious causes of endometrial bleeding must be considered. Sometimes heavy vaginal bleeding can be symptomatic of cervical, endometrial, or uterine cancer. Excessive uterine bleeding can also be caused by an IUD or by uterine fibroids.

Fibroids

Uterine fibroids are very common and most women will have some degree of this benign uterine growth during their lifetime. Uterine fibroids are non-cancerous tumors in the uterus made up of smooth muscle cells and connective tissue. While some stay very small, others can cause the uterus to stretch to the size of a five or six-month-pregnant womb. Fibroids often grow during pregnancy, and even more commonly, toward the end of the woman's reproductive life. It is generally believed that excessive estrogen promotes fibroid growth, but since they are benign many women choose to do nothing unless the fibroids cause heavy bleeding or pressure on the bowel or bladder. A small fibroid measures less than 4 cm in diameter, and I have found that small ones can be readily reduced by an anti-estrogenic diet (no animal products) and acupuncture. Medium-sized fibroids (4-10 cm) are a little tougher to treat but can certainly be reduced non-surgically. Fibroids larger than 10 cm are not easy to reduce by dietary measures alone.

Consult a qualified healthcare professional if you have more than two very heavy periods in a short time span. You will need a pelvic ultrasound to evaluate the thickness of the endometrium (the endometrial stripe) and probably an endometrial biopsy, which is like a PAP smear, but the thin, tissue-collecting instrument goes up through the os into the uterus. If you wish to have a fibroid removed, consider a myomectomy. Also known as leiomyectomy, this procedure involves removal of the fibroid only as opposed to a hysterectomy. A growing number of gynecologic surgeons can now perform this procedure laparoscopically.

When Do I Worry About Heavy Bleeding?

Unless you are losing so much blood that you risk becoming anemic, or are extremely uncomfortable with temporarily irregular menses, know that it is *normal* to have weird periods for several years before complete cessation of menses. You need to figure out what you want for yourself, and seek help accordingly. For example, some women are attached to their cycles, and want to continue bleeding regularly. This will be especially true of healthy women in their forties who have not borne any children, yet aren't ready to let go of the idea of becoming biological mothers. Healthy older moms can confer many benefits to their offspring, but the chances of an uncomplicated pregnancy diminish with age.

For women who wish to regularize their cycles, progesterone taken in the luteal phase may do the trick nicely. Older women who conceive while supplementing with progesterone are advised to continue with progesterone supplementation well into the second trimester of the pregnancy because progesterone withdrawal is the main cause of endometrial shedding (menstruation).

If heavy bleeding turns out to be from precancerous cells in the uterine lining, a short course of progesterone may be curative. Another option for controlling heavy bleeding caused by benign or precancerous endometrial proliferation is a procedure called endometrial ablation. Performed by a gynecologist or occasionally by a general surgeon, endometrial ablation involves placing an electrical device called a hysteroscope into the uterus and applying heat to destroy the endometrial lining. The heat source may involve a balloon filled with hot water, laser, or electricity. Fifty percent of the women who have this procedure never menstruate again. Less radical is the D and C, which stands for diletage (dilating the cervical os) and curretage (scraping the lining with a curved blade). A hysterectomy is usually needed for uterine or endometrial cancer.

What If I'm Not Ready to Stop Bleeding?

For women who have not menstruated for several months, but have a history of normal menstruation, a progesterone push is prescribed by the doctor. The usual prescription is 10 mg of Provera for five days, or if the doctor prefers natural hormones, 200–400 mg of oral micronized progesterone (OMP) for ten days. If the latter is prescribed, be sure it is plant-based United States Pharmacopeia (USP) progesterone (United States Pharmacopeia refers to an official reference book that lists standardized potency, naturally based, medicinal products). If progesterone is taken for the prescribed time and a period occurs within the following ten days, the hormonal function is basically intact and just needs a little help. Occasionally a young woman without regular menses will be in premature ovarian failure, or she may not have enough body fat (20 percent is needed) to menstruate. The herb *Vitex agnus castus,* taken continuously throughout the month, can effectively enhance the luteinizing hormone; remember, the LH surge triggers ovulation, which triggers progesterone production. Conventional doctors will often offer women a birth control pill if she is clearly premenopausal and wants to make her periods more regular. I don't recommend this approach because the pill contains synthetic hormones and packs a large dose of them. Even the so-called low-dose pills like Alesse contain four times more synthetic hormone than Prempro, the standard menopausal drug combination of estrogen (from horse urine) and progestins. The pill often causes digestive problems, particularly gallbladder disease, increased moodiness, and weight gain, and should be a last resort when used to stabilize hormonal fluctuations. If you smoke, have liver disease, or most important, have a personal or family history of strokes or forming blood clots, estrogen in any form is contraindicated for you because of the danger of exacerbating these health issues. Some birth control pills contain only progestins, but most contain both estrogen and progestins.

Plant Estrogens Can Help Weird Periods

Another approach to easing irregular periods, which is usually a problem of estrogen dominance, is to ingest natural phytoestrogens. These are plants (phyto) that contain estrogen-mimicking substances that can bind to estrogen receptors in our bodies, blocking them from absorbing excess estrogen. When phytoestrogens bind to estrogen receptors, the result is reduced impact from estrogen secreted from the ovaries. Such herbs therefore reduce the potentially harmful effects of the stronger estrogens (both natural and synthetic) by competing for estrogen receptor sites. These low-potency estrogenic substances include coumestans (from alfalfa), diosgenin (from wild yam), and isoflavones (from soy). Some of the signs and symptoms of estrogen excess in perimenopause that may call for the use of phytoestrogens include breast tenderness, cyclic headaches, cystic breasts and ovaries, depression, excessive uterine bleeding, fluid retention, nausea, prolonged periods, sleep disturbances, uterine fibroids, and weight gain.

While excess estrogen is the predominant cause of irregular periods and can be tempered by regular use of phytoestrogens such as alfalfa, black cohosh, licorice, red clover, soy, and wild yam, other causes must be considered. For example, heavy menstrual bleeding is a classic sign of low thyroid function. Maybe you have several more years of menstruation ahead, but your periods are getting heavier and closer together. You may simply need some thyroid support. If this is confirmed by lab tests or a thyroid-oriented clinical exam (see Chapter 19 on the thyroid), start by increasing high-iodine foods, such as fish and sea vegetables, in the diet. Avoid raw cruciferous vegetables, including bok choy, broccoli, cabbage, cauliflower, and turnips, because they can block iodine uptake by the thyroid gland.

Besides thyroid or ovarian hormone function, poor liver function, obesity, and stress can contribute to menstrual changes, including excessively heavy or irregularly spaced periods. To aid the liver, avoid drugs and stimulants, including caffeine, and have at least one daily bowel movement. If you are not eliminating regularly, increase your water and fiber intake. My favorite fiber supplement is three tablespoons of freshly ground flaxseeds stirred into juice or water. B vitamins may help with liver detoxification, especially vitamin B_6 (150 mg daily). The B vitamins are also great stress-busters, along with extra calcium and magnesium, and plenty of vitamin C (2,000 mg daily or more).

Polycystic Ovary Syndrome

An increasingly common cause of irregular periods is polycystic ovary syndrome (PCOS). Not only estrogen, but also progesterone, testosterone, and insulin may run high in PCOS. The high hormone levels cause a cluster of eggs to compete for ovulation, causing multiple small benign cysts to form around the edge of the ovary which prevent any single egg from maturing properly. Often, but not always, women with PCOS have difficulty conceiving because they are not ovulating. In fact, PCOS is one of the most common causes of female infertility in the United States. The high insulin levels present in PCOS may be accompanied by high levels of blood glucose and high triglycerides. The syndrome is related to Syndrome X, which is a bit like diabetes. In both Syndrome X and PCOS the problem is insulin resistance, where the cells are no longer sensitive to insulin and therefore do not allow for insulin uptake. Since insulin is required in order to facilitate sugar uptake into the cells from the bloodstream, levels of sugar (glucose) in the blood become dangerously high without it. Excess sugar in the blood is like rust—first it insidiously erodes the insides of blood vessels, and then, ultimately, the organs, especially the ones with the most blood, such as the backs of the eyes, the kidneys, the ovaries, and the thyroid gland.

Another common symptom of PCOS is male-pattern hair growth, such as facial hair growth and lots of hair on the limbs. Many women with PCOS can be helped by a precise hormone analysis and subsequent hormone balancing, and by controlling their blood-sugar levels, preferably through diet, but they may need medication. Instead of balking at a commitment to a lower carbohydrate (low-sugar) diet, first think about what yummy things you *can* eat: avocados, macadamia and other nuts, olives, olive oil, and salmon. Commercially produced baked goods (all breads, cakes, cookies, pies, and so on) need to be eliminated from the diet, slowly but surely.

Spotting

Spotting between periods can be annoying or worrisome. Spotting is usually not a scary problem, although a PAP smear and possibly a pelvic ultrasound are important tests to rule out cervical or uterine cancer as the source of the spotting. If spotting occurs after intercourse, the cause may sometimes be a benign cervical polyp, which bleeds easily from friction. Your local gynecologist or internist should be able to perform a minor surgical procedure to remove the polyp.

Spotting between periods, especially when the spotting occurs around mid-cycle, is often a result of reduced progesterone levels. The endometrium is not as readily retained and starts to drip before the actual monthly flow. Occasionally mid-cycle spotting can actually mean a pregnancy, because implantation bleeding is not uncommon. Some women will actually have a normal period two weeks after an embryo has been implanted. Know whether or not you are pregnant before doing anything drastic such as acupuncture, diet, exercise, herbs, or other treatments to deal with mid-cycle spotting. If you're not pregnant, chaste tree berry (also called vitex from the Latin name *Vitex agnus castus*) can promote progesterone and improve the spotting problem. Work with a qualified herbalist or alternative practitioner to determine dosing specifics.

Endometriosis: Extremely Painful Bleeding

If your bleeding is especially heavy, prolonged, and painful, you may have a condition called endometriosis, which is caused by displaced uterine tissue also bleeding during the menstrual period. The most common place for ectopic (outside the normal place) uterine tissue (endometrium) is around the ovaries, because the endometrium improperly migrates through the fallopian tubes and clusters at the ends of the tubes where the ovaries are located. Improper migration of the endometrial tissue may be caused by pressure in the vagina or uterus, such as from intercourse during menstruation, tampon use, or even prolonged inverted poses (such as hanging from gravity boots) while menstruating. Menstruating women attending yoga classes are always advised to avoid doing headstands and shoulder stands if they are bleeding heavily. If you suspect endometriosis, avoid sex and tampons during your period.

Cures for endometriosis include laparoscopic surgery and cauterization of the ectopic tissue so it no longer bleeds. It may also be possible to work with natural methods, such as hormone balancing, pain control, styptic (to control bleeding) herbs such as capsella bursa-pastoris (shepherd's purse) and diet to resolve this cause of painful menstruation. Some doctors consider endometriosis to be an autoimmune disease and apply therapies to minimize inappropriate immune reactions. Pregnancy can sometimes cure endometriosis.

Estrogens in Commercial Meat Must Be Avoided

Excess estrogen plays a role in endometriosis, as well as other problematic menstrual presentations, and avoiding estrogen sources in the diet is a great place to start healing. By far, chicken is the very highest source of estrogen in commercially available food, so use hormone-free, organically raised, range-fed chickens whenever possible. Don't eat chicken in a restaurant unless they specialize in all organic food. In certain parts of the United States, particularly in Hispanic populations along the Texas border with Mexico, precocious puberty is endemic. Girls as young as age eight are menstruating and developing breasts. These findings correlate with increased chicken consumption there.

Anyone who needs further convincing about the perils of eating chicken might want to peruse the works of John Robbins. His first book, and video, *Diet for a New America,* was a real eye-opener for me. He recently came out with another book, *Food Revolution,* which is compelling reading for those who want to live in a way that supports both the health of their bodies and the planet as a whole. Another shocker is *Fast Food Nation* by Eric Schlosser, which is a meticulously detailed history of the fast food industry. Animal flesh and animal byproducts such as milk and cheese are the most important sources of excessive, and usually harmful, estrogen in our diets. Avoid commercial red meat and chicken whenever possible, and try to get multiple servings of fresh fruits and vegetables daily.

Coffee is a widely overlooked source of estrogen-like substances that derive from the pesticides sprayed on South American coffee crops. Coffee beans are naturally oily, and thus absorb toxins more readily than fibrous, water-soluble foods. Of all crops, coffee, along with cacao (chocolate) and avocados receive the heaviest pesticide treatment because bugs love them, too. Try to use organically produced varieties of these crops whenever possible. Be aware that what you put into your mouth provides the building blocks for cellular repair and hormone production, and keeps you a fully functioning, well-balanced, healthy being. Keep it clean.

Achieve and Maintain Your Optimum Weight

Try to achieve your appropriate weight. I like to figure a good ballpark weight by calculating the BMI, or basal metabolic index. Take your weight in pounds and multiply by 703. Then, take your height in inches, and square that number. The weight number will be larger. Divide it by the height number. This gives you another number, usually in the 20s, which is your BMI. A good BMI falls between 19 and 25. A number below 19 is too thin; higher than 25 is starting to get too heavy. A BMI greater than 30 is considered obese. For example, I am 5' 7" (67 inches) tall and weight 130 pounds. The weight (130 x 703 = 91390) divided by the height (67 x 67 = 4489) is 20.38. That's about 20, an optimal BMI. Another quick check for appropriate, healthy weight is waist size. Ladies: 34 inches should be the max! (For men, it's 40 inches max, but optimally no more than 38 inches.)

A Typical Set of Premenopausal Symptoms

Carol, a forty-six-year-old woman, had a job she loved, grown children, and a comfortable home and marriage, but when she came to see me she said she was falling apart at the seams. For the past two years, her periods had been unpredictable. She would go for months without one and start thinking she was done with menstruation. Then, out of the blue she'd have a really heavy period which would be, needless to say, worse than a bad hair day. On top of that, she said she felt vaguely anxious and had difficulty thinking clearly, especially in the afternoon, and wasn't sleeping well. After further questioning I ascertained that her poor sleep was mostly because of temperature fluctuations—she'd feel chilly at bedtime, then would suddenly get a heat surge and throw off the bed covers during the night. She also told me that her heavy periods were accompanied by painful breast tenderness (a classic symptom of too much estrogen). So, what did I diagnose? You got it—waning progesterone and an excess of estrogen. Simply put, Carol was perimenopausal.

As women age, they are increasingly likely to have anovulatory cycles, which are menstrual cycles where no ovulation occurs. When a woman such as Carol doesn't ovulate, she doesn't produce the progesterone that ultimately helps to shed the uterine lining. Perimenopausal women like her are likely to have several anovulatory cycles in a row; then, when a chance ovulation does occur (after all, the hormones are still cycling), the blood that has built up over several months will gush out once the progesterone drops off. Anxiety, foggy thinking, night sweats, and sleep disturbances are all well-documented results of progesterone deficiency. Since Carol was ready to stop menstruating, the prescription for her was a low-dose natural progesterone (100 mg OMP–oral micronized progesterone) daily, with a week off every first week of the month. She followed my instructions and was back to feeling like her old self in no time at all.

Making days one through seven of each month drug-free is simply for the convenience of remembering the protocol for women no longer menstruating regularly. If this lapse of one week monthly begins to produce more regular menses, and this is not desired, use less progesterone (50 mg, or the minimal amount to control symptoms—this will vary with the individual woman) on a continuous basis. Cyclic (not continuous) progesterone use is helpful for younger women who are having weird periods and want to resume a more normal pattern.

Treatment Summary

❋ Progesterone (be sure to use plant-based USP progesterone), 100 mg daily in the second half of the menstrual cycle, may help restore regularity to the menstrual flow.

❋ *Vitex agnus castus* (a medicinal berry, also known as chaste tree berry because it was once given to monks to reduce their libido) taken all month long can be very effective in normalizing periods and smoothing out fluctuating hormones. Work with a qualified herbalist or naturopathic doctor to find a good source of vitex and figure out the right dose for you.

❋ Eat plant (phyto) estrogens, such as soy products. Potent substances, such as hormones, get into cells through a keyhole (cell receptors) where they then turn on specific activity within the cells, such as making more hormones. The plant estrogens fit into the keyhole, but just sit there and don't trigger estrogen type activities in the cell. Since most perimenopausal problems are caused by too much estrogen, eating plant estrogens will block the excess circulating estrogen from getting into the cells. The best forms of soy to eat (in terms of effectiveness in blocking estrogen) are miso (one tablespoon daily), tofu (one-quarter block daily), or soy nuts (a tasty, crunchy snack, sort of like corn nuts, one-half cup daily). Use organic soy products to avoid GMO ingestion.

❋ *Capsella bursa-pastoris* (shepherd's purse) is a potent styptic (stanches blood flow). For heavy menstrual bleeds, capsella can slow things down so the blood loss is not so scary. It also works well for nosebleeds. However, if you have very heavy menstruation, see a doctor, preferably a gynecologist, as soon as possible, since a serious problem like endometrial cancer must be ruled out.

❋ It is important to achieve and maintain your optimum weight. Aim for a BMI (basal metabolic index) under 25.

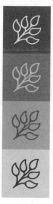

2.

Mood Swings— Even My Dog Notices

here is a widely held belief that all women are unpredictably moody because of hormonal imbalances. You've all heard the jokes and nasty digs about how women can get catty before their periods. Don't buy it. This bad propaganda about all women is depressing enough, but it's even worse given the realities of a woman in midlife who is likely to be juggling several jobs and family responsibilities every single day. (If you check the medical literature, the prevalence of depression and moodiness is actually much higher in younger women.) The incidence of depression in women peaks during childbearing years and decreases after age forty-five. Interviews from doctors' practices in Holland on nearly 9,000 women and men aged twenty-five to seventy-five showed *no* gender differences in moodiness or depression. Interestingly, women who undergo surgical menopause (a hysterectomy) have higher depression rates than women anticipating or experiencing natural menopause.

On the other hand, I challenge you to find an American woman who hasn't experienced some degree of PMS (premenstrual syndrome) in herself or a close friend or relative. Those three little letters have added up to some pretty huge disruptions of personal, family, and professional routines. They are arguably one reason we have yet to bring to office a female President of the United States (although I have no doubt that milestone will be achieved).

The ABCDs of PMS

Premenstrual syndrome encompasses four basic categories of disturbances that occur before the monthly bleeding and are very much propelled by hormonal fluctuations. The four types of PMS are:

- PMS-A (anxiety and irritability)

- PMS-B (bloating)

- PMS-C (cravings for certain foods, increased appetite)

- PMS-D (depression and insomnia)

Most women who have PMS will experience symptoms from more than one group, but PMS-A is the most common type. The anxiety, irritability, and nervous tension that rise to a frenetic crescendo between ovulation and menses are evocative of the extreme mood swings often experienced in peri-menopause, when the hormones are trying to go through their monthly changes while also dealing with a much bigger change as the ovaries run out of eggs. Same pesky problem: fewer ovulations means less progesterone, and relatively higher levels of estrogen. Progesterone is a potent antidepressant. Estrogen excess provokes irritability. Keep in mind that in perimenopause, the first phase of menopause, testosterone is the last hormone to wane, making the irritability of estrogen excess even more aggressive. Although I have never seen research specifically devoted to the topic, I would speculate that women who have experienced the more severe symptoms of PMS are more likely to have a bumpier ride through the perimenopausal phase. Take heart, though. There is much you can do to manage your menopause naturally and smooth out the road ahead. While herbs and progesterone may help, I'd like to go into more detail about a therapeutic lifestyle featuring a health-promoting diet and a healthy outlook.

Get to Know Yourself

The most important relationship in life is the one with self. Various cultures throughout human history, particularly cultures consciously living in har-mony with nature such as agrarian societies, have defined the phases of a woman's life by her ability to bear children. Using this viewpoint the first phase is maiden, the second phase is mother, and the third phase is matriarch. When you visualize someone with older-woman status, get past the stereo-types and consider the feisty older woman who wears purple and wide-brimmed hats, sings for any occasion, prepares delicious feasts, loves to explore and travel, and is still very lively despite the dearth of eggs in her ovaries. This lively older woman may not have thick long hair or perfectly smooth skin, but she adds a great deal to her community in terms of volunteer service or a high level of professional productivity that comes with long experience, or simply through the good cheer that comes from her decision to embrace life fully. And as the responsibilities of tending to children and parents have likely lessened, she probably has the time and financial security to explore herself as never before. These are good changes. For those of us struggling through the harrowing pitfalls of approaching menopause, let us begin with the realization that with a little imagination, forethought, and dedication we will emerge victorious, having attained the bliss of older-woman/matriarchal status.

Daily Fun Factor

Plan to engage in some activity that you really *want* to do every day—not just those you should do, or have to do, or need to do. It would hardly be worth getting out of bed for a day full of "shoulds," would it? Hopefully, the activity you really want to do will also promote your health and well-being. For example, you can find a fun form of physical exercise. Or meet a girlfriend for a get-together over tea. Or indulge in a nice long session with your journal. Here's another idea: try meditation. Most communities have a teaching center for learning and practicing basic meditation techniques, which involve conscious breathing. You can start there, in a comfortable position, allowing the diaphragm to rise and fall with the breath, breathing through the nose only if possible, making the exhalation at least as long as the inhalation, and allowing the breath to become deeper and more drawn out as you continue. A warm bath is always good for improving your mood, especially if you can get all set up with epsom salts (two big handfuls of this readily available form of magnesium, nature's prime muscle relaxant), soft music and candles, and maybe a cup of tea. If you enjoy sweating, find a steam room or sauna in your community that you can use. Maybe you even know how to participate in sweat lodges. Just let that irritation that has built up come right out of your pores. Walking helps almost any moody funk. Make it a regular practice, especially if you have access to sites of natural beauty. Sometimes just sitting and relaxing quietly in the dark, as a form of meditation, can help bring perspective.

Any of these activities will add pleasure to your day and reduce the tension and stress that women may be susceptible to at this time in life. Remember, these mood swings are temporary, and you don't want to incur permanent damage to yourself or to important relationships in a fit of rage. Think about people and places you love. Contemplate peaceful images, and explore the possibility of forgiveness of yourself and others.

Nerve Nutrients

At a physiological level, there are many natural agents, including herbal medicines, that can promote a deeper sense of well-being and help you weather the storms of estrogen-induced mood swings. The B vitamins (B_6 in particular) are nerve nutrients, and the mineral magnesium, as mentioned above, is my favorite natural muscle relaxant. For those who tend toward depression as well as moodiness the amino acid tryptophan will promote serotonin levels, which typically enhances a feeling of well-being. I recommend tryptophan in its precursor form, 5-HTP (5-hydroxy-tryptophan), because lower doses are required.

A good night's sleep is the ultimate panacea—we have all experienced how much better we feel after seven to eight solid hours of deep slumber. 5-hydroxy-tryptophan can be taken at bedtime (50–300 mg, but start at the lower dose) to produce more restful sleep, and its benefit as a mild antidepressant will carry over into the next day. Melatonin (I like low doses—0.5 mg at bedtime) is another safe, effective sleep aid.

Helpful Herbs

Herbal medicines, taken in liquid form as teas or alcohol extractions or as the whole plant, dried, crushed, and placed in capsules, are still used as the primary tools for universal ailments in 75 percent of the world. The following list of herbs fall into a category called nervines: plant medicines that soothe the central nervous system. This list is far from complete, but can provide a springboard for further exploration of this safe, effective, and quintessentially natural form of self-care.

- Black cohosh (*Cimicifuga racemosa*) is very effective for reducing hot flashes.

- Catnip (*Nepeta cataria*), not just for cats, has a soothing aromatic oil.

- Chamomile (*Matricaria recucita*) is not just for children. While it is best known for its soothing and sedative effect, a strong brew is mildly stimulating.

- Dong quai (*Angelica sinensis*). Chewing the root relieves cramps quickly.

- Flaxseed (*Linum usitatissimum*). Ingested, the fresh oil prevents inflammation.

- Hops (*Humulus lupulus*) (the flavoring in many beers) is a relaxant, despite raising prolactin levels.

- Lemon balm (*Melissa officinalis*) is one of my favorite herbs for nervous stomach.

- Oats (*Avena sativa*). Stuff into a clean sock, then run your bathwater through it and allow the mildly sedative qualities to soak in as you bathe.

- Passionflower (*Passiflora incarnata*) works for nerve pain.

- Eleutherococcus (*Eleutherococcus senticosus*) works well to increase white blood cells. (This herb is also known as Siberian ginseng.)

- Skullcap (*Scutellaria laterifolia*) is especially useful for moodiness with constipation.

- St. John's wort (*Hypericum perforatum*) is excellent for moderate depression.

- Valerian (*Valeriana officinalis*) is an effective analgesic (pain-reducer).

Food and Mood

When you are trying to reduce the effect of estrogen on your mood, intake of the following foods should be minimized because they promote estrogen levels. First and most significant are animal products. The others may surprise you: alfalfa, apples, barley, brown rice, carrots, cherries, coconut, nightshade family (eggplant, peppers, potatoes, tobacco, tomatoes), olives, peanuts, plums, soy products, wheat, and yams. Avoid all fried, processed, and refined foods.

Choose organic produce whenever possible, keeping in mind that organic produce means you're not getting the pesticide residues that can make any food a health liability. Mixing ingredients for a gourmet meal is fine, but train yourself to snack only on whole foods, meaning a food that stands alone, such as a piece of fruit or a vegetable—something that was growing not too long ago. One of my nutrition teachers used to say, "Don't eat anything that wouldn't rot, but eat it before it does."

Figuring out ahead of time what you're going to eat tomorrow will dramatically improve the chances of your food choices being healthy. I'd like to share some tips on making healthy choices on a day-to-day basis, forever. I take time on a weekend day to make two lists: one is lunch and dinner meals for the coming week, and the other is a grocery list for the ingredients I don't have on hand to accomplish my week's menus. I'll often make two big pots of soup or stew to freeze in meal-sized containers for the days ahead. This may seem tedious while grinding through the task, but it makes life flow a lot more smoothly in the week to come.

Movement Is a Must

Another crucial lifestyle choice that will greatly enhance healthy longevity is regular, moderate exercise. Don't wear yourself out. However, some kind of daily vigorous movement is a panacea that is almost as important as sleep. I know for myself that if I don't include exercise sessions in my schedule, they are less likely to occur. Anything that involves work rarely happens spontaneously on a regular basis, even something that can be fun, like exercise. Some prefer to exercise alone, or a group setting may work better for you. Consider inviting a buddy to join you on a regular basis. In China, women and men traditionally begin their daily practice of tai chi chu'an in their mid-to-late fifties to maintain their energy levels and good joint flexibility. It is never too late to start a regular exercise program, but the sooner the better.

Your Future Is Under Your Control

Your well-being in this glorious later phase of your life will be greatly enhanced by good health, a positive outlook, a sense of belonging, and a general sense of satisfaction with life. All these factors are within your control if you make a commitment to help yourself. Don't fall into the trap of believing that menopause is a disease requiring medication. Too much drug advertising portrays the older woman as anxious and decrepit, as nothing but a burden to society until she can restore her life through drugs. Ironically, improper use of prescription medications is the fourth leading cause of death in the United States (after heart disease, cancer, and the complications of obesity).

Many older women are enjoying life more than ever, and you owe it to yourself to have a great life, too. For many women, life really begins anew after the years of dedication to career and family. Stay focused on these bright possibilities while doing what you can to mitigate the vagaries of violently fluctuating moods. This phase will pass.

Treatment Summary

❀ Are you feeling outraged and out-of-control again? Try to keep the reassuring fact in mind that this is a passing phase. You will *not* be like this forever. Try to take time out for yourself as soon as possible.

❀ Take time out for yourself *every day*. It is vitally important to have time alone, without the pressure of having to accomplish a task, if only for twenty minutes a day. Lock yourself in the bathroom to take a bubble bath and read a novel. I'm sure you can figure out what would work for you. Make it happen.

❀ Vitamin B_6 is one of my favorite nerve soothers. Doses up to 250 mg daily can work wonders, especially in the premenstrual time. You can't overdose on B vitamins because they are water-soluble and excess amounts will be excreted. The smallest effective dose is always advisable, however, so if high doses help, work down to lower doses to find the lowest that works as well. You may only need 30–50 mg daily, but supplement with a B-complex to make it more effective (the B vitamins work better when taken together).

❀ Magnesium is excellent as a muscle and brain relaxant. You can take liquid or capsule supplements at bedtime, up to 1,000 mg. Start with 150 mg because magnesium can give you loose bowel movements. Taking magnesium at bedtime will help you get a good night's sleep, which always makes the next day go better. You can also add two double handfuls of epsom salts (magnesium sulfate) to your bathwater and the magnesium will absorb right through your skin.

❀ Herbal nervines, plant medicines that soothe the central nervous system, are safe and effective. Try them.

❀ Avoid all animal products—dairy products (especially cheese, milk, and ice cream) and meat—because they are high in estrogen.

❀ Regular moderate exercise is important for enhancing your health and graceful aging.

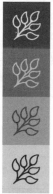

3.

Breast Tenderness—
Ouch! Don't Hug Me

Although water retention is not a very common symptom of perimenopause, it can really be a beast for the women who experience
breast tenderness. Some women complain that they cannot bear to
be even lightly hugged, or lie face down. Some can't even endure the weight
of water from the shower hitting their breasts. Believe it or not, women with
smaller breasts tend to be more prone to this problem because their breast tissue is more densely compacted, without much stretch potential for periods of
expansion. Breast tissue is complex; much of it is fibrous or fatty and riddled
with ducts (to carry the milk to the nipple), lobules (to hold the fat cells), and
fluid-filled cysts. Hormones are fat-based molecules and can be easily stored
in fatty tissues such as the breasts. Tender breasts can result from an excess of
estrogen, progesterone, or aldosterone, the most active of the adrenal secretions and the one that regulates sodium, chloride, and potassium metabolism.
Women prone to generalized fluid retention, including monthly weight gain,
swollen ankles, abdomen, and face, will be particularly helped by addressing
any excess of aldosterone. It may seem counterintuitive, but one approach to
increased water weight is to drink plenty of water. This will dilute the minerals that are holding the excess fluid inside the cells. Some researchers believe
it is the confluence of all three of these hormones in excess that causes this
particular symptom. While breast tenderness is not related to increased rates
of breast disease, persistent breast pain, particularly if it is in one breast only,
must be evaluated by a health professional as soon as possible.

Listen Up, Chocoholics!

If you haven't already figured out that caffeinated sodas, chocolate, and coffee (and for some, even black tea) make breast tenderness worse, take note. There is strong evidence documenting an association between consumption of these beverages, all containing methylxanthines (caffeine, theobromine, and theophylline) and the stimulation of fibrous tissue and cystic fluid. One study of women who limited their methylxanthine intake showed a nearly 98 percent improvement in breast tenderness.

The Miracle of Vitamin E

Women with more fibrous, dense breasts may have more hormone receptors in their breast tissue, which would account for their breast tissue being denser. More hormone receptors means more hormonal activity, with a resulting increase of bloating in the fluid-holding areas of the breasts (the cystic and fibrous areas) and an increased sensitization by hormones in the fatty areas. Besides replacing your caffeine and colas with water, I have found vitamin E to be very useful for treating breast engorgement. Most women with significant breast tenderness related to hormonal changes need 1,200–1,600 IU (international units) daily to solve the problem. As your hormones settle down after menopause, the breast tenderness should disappear, or be mitigated by avoiding methylxanthines and using a maintenance dose of 400–800 IU vitamin E daily. Consult with a qualified practitioner of nutritional medicine to find a good vitamin E product in your area. Many manufacturers, unfortunately, cheat on vitamin E production, as it is relatively more expensive to produce and keep stable than the water-soluble vitamins, such as the Bs and C. No one cheats on making the B or C vitamins because they can be produced inexpensively. I personally endorse the use of vitamin E products from J.R. Carlson Laboratories of Arlington Heights, Illinois.

Along with A, D, and K, vitamin E is one of the fat-soluble vitamins and it is generally processed from soybean oil. When choosing a vitamin E product, look for d-alpha, the natural form, rather than the synthetic dl-alpha. Some nutritionists prefer vitamin E in a base of mixed tocopherols (which includes the delta and gamma fractions of the molecule), claiming this mix provides more antioxidant action than d-alpha alone, but I have been very happy with the d-alpha Carlson products I have used in my practice for more than fifteen years. (See Chapter 14 for more information on vitamin E.) If you are diagnosed with breast cancer, know that the "dry" vitamin E in the succinate form has been shown to be more effective than d-alpha in preventing recurrence after treatment.

Too Much Estrogen

If your breast tenderness is getting worse and you have taken the appropriate measures (breast exam by a professional, a mammogram, and an ultrasound) to make sure no breast disease exists, estrogen dominance is a likely culprit and supplemental progesterone may help. Do not use synthetic progestins, as all the new evidence points to progestins being problematic for breast tissue. Work with an experienced healthcare provider to determine the best form and dose of progesterone for you.

If you take a birth control pill, which contains much higher levels of hormones (including progestins in many types of oral contraceptives) than the HRT (hormone replacement therapy) levels, switch to fertility awareness or the cervical cap. Fertility awareness involves carefully tracking the signs of your ovulation—a soft, high cervix with slippery egg-white cervical mucus—and avoiding sex that would allow sperm to contact the cervix up to five days before predicted ovulation. It's OK for teenage girls who are sexually active to use the pill to prevent an unwanted pregnancy, but for older and theoretically more mature adults, barrier methods or abstinence at ovulation are examples of contraceptive methods that are friendlier to your body than the pill. A higher incidence of breast cancer has been correlated with pill use by women in their forties—again, probably due more to the progestin than the estrogen component.

Or Maybe It's Too Much Progesterone

Sometimes breast tenderness gets worse after women begin using the very popular and widely available progesterone creams. If this happens, it should tip you off that excess progesterone might be the problem. I've seen numerous saliva hormone results showing progesterone levels that are way off the chart due to supplemental use. Some practitioners claim that topical progesterone (or any hormone) is so well absorbed through the skin that much lower doses can be used effectively because these hormones go directly into the bloodstream, avoiding the first pass through the liver that occurs when substances enter our bodies via the mouth. This may be true, and certainly anything ingested is processed with stomach acid, mixed with bile and pancreatic enzymes and digested before it goes into the blood. Food-based molecules are generally considered friendly (and therefore readily accepted) by our internal environment; however, I personally prefer to use oral hormone supplementation in my practice because dosing is more easily monitored and adjusted.

Or Maybe a Kidney Problem

If you are getting bloated all over, you may have a kidney problem, and not just a temporary hormonally related fluid-balance problem. Sodium restriction may help with a tendency to hold water weight, but see a doctor if the problem persists. My favorite herbal medicine to cleanse both the kidneys and the liver, and to act as a deep but gentle diuretic, is the humble dandelion plant. *Taraxacum officinales* grows nearly everywhere in the United States and is mostly considered a weed, but the root of the plant is particularly potent as a diuretic, and it is rich in potassium, unlike many of the prescription diuretics (such as Lasix) which are very difficult to wean off once started. If you know anyone taking a prescription diuretic, let them know that they should supplement with 100 mg of potassium daily. Dandelion leaves are also organ cleansers and perhaps less diuretic. The French nickname for dandelion is pis-en-lit, which means wet your bed. (Country mothers know to not feed their young children dandelion greens at suppertime.) Our word for this healing plant comes from the French dents-de-lion, which means lion's teeth, and refers to the deep, tooth-like indentations along the edges of the leaves.

Soothing Castor Oil Packs

One final treatment tip for tender, fibrocystic breasts is the topical application of castor oil and heat. Castor oil packs are one of my favorite naturopathic tools, and they help many congestive conditions including constipation, hepatitis, joint sprains, painful menstruation, and more. You can buy bottles of castor oil (nicknamed palma Christi, or the hand of Christ) at most drugstores, and follow the instructions on the label. For ease of use, I prefer to use castor oil in a roll-on form (like a deodorant stick), and I get mine from Gen MacManiman, in Fall City, Washington. I consider a castor oil roll-on an essential part of any home first-aid kit, along with Arnica cream or gel (for soft tissue trauma, especially bruises), some form of magnesium (for cramps or sore muscles), hydrogen peroxide (for cleaning wounds), and Rescue Remedy (a combination of flower extractions created by Edward Bach, which is very effective for soothing ruffled emotions). At the first sign of breast tenderness, apply castor oil to the breast and cover with plastic wrap, then a heating pad for at least twenty minutes. Do this daily for a week or until the breast tenderness is resolved.

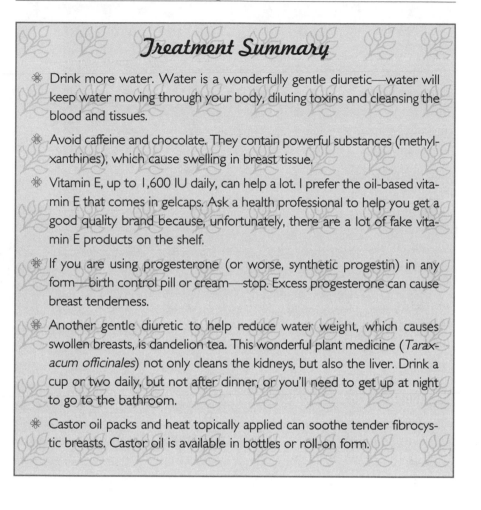

Treatment Summary

❋ Drink more water. Water is a wonderfully gentle diuretic—water will keep water moving through your body, diluting toxins and cleansing the blood and tissues.

❋ Avoid caffeine and chocolate. They contain powerful substances (methyl-xanthines), which cause swelling in breast tissue.

❋ Vitamin E, up to 1,600 IU daily, can help a lot. I prefer the oil-based vitamin E that comes in gelcaps. Ask a health professional to help you get a good quality brand because, unfortunately, there are a lot of fake vitamin E products on the shelf.

❋ If you are using progesterone (or worse, synthetic progestin) in any form—birth control pill or cream—stop. Excess progesterone can cause breast tenderness.

❋ Another gentle diuretic to help reduce water weight, which causes swollen breasts, is dandelion tea. This wonderful plant medicine (*Taraxacum officinales*) not only cleans the kidneys, but also the liver. Drink a cup or two daily, but not after dinner, or you'll need to get up at night to go to the bathroom.

❋ Castor oil packs and heat topically applied can soothe tender fibrocystic breasts. Castor oil is available in bottles or roll-on form.

4.

No Sex Drive— Is This Permanent?

Just when the kids are starting to take up less of your time and your body isn't in constant demand by someone else, and the idea of romance seems like a possibility again . . . no sex drive.

Libido is a complex topic. There are numerous reasons your sex drive may be low, including coexisting medical problems, reduced vaginal lubrication, side effects of drugs (a major reason), and perhaps changes in your relationship with your mate. Some women find the years approaching menopause (when the likelihood of pregnancy becomes increasingly remote) very exciting, sexually and otherwise. If you are among them and your sex life is terrific, you probably won't feel compelled to read this chapter.

It can be difficult to approach the topic of sex with a doctor, especially if the doctor typically spends little time with you and is not particularly warm and fuzzy. Female doctors are likely to be more approachable, but their gender is certainly not a guarantee of warm fuzziness, so it depends on the individual doctor. There are numerous physical changes induced by hormonal changes, which will be discussed below, but first let's consider the mind, arguably the most erogenous center of one's being.

Close Your Eyes, Take a Deep Breath

You must ask yourself, in a quiet, unhurried setting, "Do I still like my mate?" If the answer is a clear "Yes," the libido will be easier to fix. If you and your mate have grown apart it will be difficult to find closeness through sex alone. If you are committed to your mate for now, because of children, finances, or habit, you can work toward better communication skills and more emphasis on loving feelings together, or with the help of a marriage or sex counselor.

Divorce rates are higher than ever, which raises the question of whether life-long monogamy is truly natural to the human species. Some claim that men tend to be polygamous (the seed-spreading line of argument) whereas women tend to be monogamous (to protect the children, don't need visual variety in sex partners the way men do, and so on). The edges of these lines of thought have become blurred. With equal educational opportunities and income parity for women in the United States becoming more commonplace, differences between men and women that were previously attributed to gender may perhaps have less to do with penises and vaginas and more to do with personal power.

One trend I witness in my clinical practice, and through discussion with my colleagues, is that partners with a similar approach to life tend to stay together and have better sex than partners who drift apart because of a lack of deep common interests. For many couples the deep common interest is their progeny. Once the kids leave home, these couples may lose their main reason for staying together. Of course, they can grow together into the next phase of blissful matrimony, and that's the best solution. However, if one partner is intent on growing and the other partner is content with the current state of affairs, there is a potentially irreconcilable difference in how to approach life. My observation is that when one person is galvanized by the concept of self-actualization, and wants to learn and grow, these urges will ultimately overpower the need to stay with a more stagnated partner. This is called outgrowing your partner.

Most marriage counselors attempt to keep marriages together, since leaving something not so great for something worse is a possible consequence of divorce. Staying together is fine if each member of the couple can accept the style of their mate, and find what they need within themselves or through other friends. If it feels like your mate is holding you back, or is not supportive of what you sincerely perceive as personal development, then the conflict will increase and eventually demand some form of resolution. Meanwhile, unless sex is the glue in your relationship, it is not likely that you will be highly motivated to be intimate with a mate who is losing your interest.

Is This about Hormones?

There may be physical reasons the libido is waning, because the sex drive is very much hormonally driven. Think about it. A woman is more vulnerable, eats more, and can do less work when she's pregnant and tending to young children. Therefore pregnancy would not be a particularly desirable state, from a sexual standpoint, unless the results were spectacular, which of course they are.

I can't help but wonder at what point in human history women became interested in orgasms, and not just in the perpetuation of the species. Certainly sex appeal is very ancient and primal, and it is broadly demonstrated in both the animal and plant kingdoms. But what about women actually enjoying sex for its sheer physical and emotional pleasure? My hunch is that the recognition and valuation of female libido and desire for sexual fulfillment is relatively new. Many of the world cultures attempting to keep women second-class citizens also deprive women of their sexual pleasure. But if the evolution of the human species includes a balance of power between the two genders, then it logically follows that women's need for sexual pleasure will prevail. It is not easy to evolve beyond our biology, because in many fundamental ways we are still animals acting in nature to secure food and genetic continuity. Moreover, the female body is equipped with a complex hormonal system that is arguably geared exclusively to the function of bearing young.

No doubt about it, estrogen not only causes an egg to drop, it also lubricates the vagina and provides tiny tracks to guide the sperm into the uterus. As estrogen wanes, the tissues of the vagina atrophy and get drier and thinner. Just when we didn't need to worry about getting pregnant anymore, intercourse may become uncomfortable. Gay women may be spared the birth control dilemmas, but like all women, they will contend with the physical effects of decreased hormone levels: more urinary tract infections, incontinence, vaginal infections, vaginal or uterine bleeding, and decreased clitoral sensation.

Lubricants

Vaginal dryness is a common problem experienced by women approaching menopause. There are several lubricating options to address this problem, including Astroglide, but I prefer a good quality (Carlson) vitamin E oil. Like all the fat-soluble vitamins, vitamin E is a prohormone. It not only provides lubrication to the vaginal area (the head of the penis makes a good applicator, if you are so inclined) but will, with regular use, help restore some plumpness to the vaginal tissues. Other lubricating products may contain low levels of mentholated substances, to provide a tingly sensation and enhance local blood flow, such as the product Viacreme, which also contains L-arginine. (You can also take 2 grams of L-arginine a day, by mouth.)

Herbal Aphrodisiacs

Low libido may initially be caused by low progesterone levels. This relates to the estrogen-dominance theory previously discussed. If you don't want to start with progesterone, both ginseng (100 mg two to three times daily) and black cohosh (40 mg daily) may enhance lubrication and stimulate arousal. A plant commonly called horny goat weed (botanical name *Epimedium grandiflorum*) works well for enhancing blood flow to the labia and clitoris, but takes sixty to ninety minutes to achieve full effect. Use a standardized product (10 percent active ingredient) at 500–1,000 mg per dose. It works!

Other traditional herbal medicines useful in promoting blood flow to the clitoris (and its counterpart, the penis) include Spanish fly (*Cantharis*), yohimbe (*pansinistalia yohimbine*), and damiana (*Damiana mexicali*). Three additional supplements are: L-arginine, which works like Viagra to increase the levels and activity of nitric oxide (NO) and sustain the erection of the clitoris; choline, which is a precursor to the nervous system's major parasympathetic neurotransmitter, acetylcholine; and vitamin B_5, which improves the endurance of genital engorgement.

Hormones or Honey?

If the herbal or nutraceutical approaches to restoring vaginal lubrication are not to your liking, you may try progesterone, either in a cyclic fashion (half of the month if you are still menstruating) or directly applied to the vaginal area before sexual activity. Progesterone supplementation will most likely be effective in the woman who is still menstruating. If your menses are erratic, or have stopped, estrogen has a well-documented positive effect on vaginal tissues, both taken internally and applied topically. Estrogen suppositories are also available, as are vitamin E suppositories. Believe it or not, honey works wonderfully to restore a lush quality to the vagina. It's a little messy, but tasty. Ask your pharmacist for an applicator (such as a wide-mouth syringe).

Of the hormone options, testosterone cream, applied topically to the clitoris and vagina, works best, but it is not much used yet. The connection between sex drive and testosterone in both men and women is well documented. However, there has been relatively little research on testosterone, which is surprising since men's interests have largely dictated the direction of scientific medical research in the past century. But then again, men needed women to stay feminine, supporting the concept that popularized estrogen supplementation as early as the 1950s. My clinical experience has shown that testosterone taken internally at doses required to produce enhanced libido for women typically also produces aggressive behavior, deepening of the voice, facial hair growth, and other potentially disturbing masculine characteristics. Sometimes hormone analysis leads me to prescribe low-dose testosterone for bone density improvement, but for the libido issue I prefer to prescribe a specially compounded testosterone cream—$\frac{1}{2}$ gram applied topically to the genital area shortly before anticipated sexual activity. Work with a doctor who uses a compounding pharmacist to find the right dose for you.

Treatment Summary

❋ Improve communication with your mate. Let him or her know what you need to keep romance in your relationship. Try writing love letters.

❋ Look at prescription medications you may be taking. Particularly notorious for killing the sex drive are antidepressants (Elavil, Prozac, Xanax, Zoloft, and others.) and heart medications (especially the beta-blockers like Atenolol and Propanalol).

❋ Try vaginal lubricants. There are some wild choices out there in a variety of flavors. I like a good quality vitamin E gel best.

❋ Herbal aphrodisiacs, black cohosh or ginseng for example, can enhance lubrication and stimulate arousal.

❋ The amino acid L-arginine, either taken internally (2 grams daily) or applied directly to the clitoral area, will enhance nitric oxide levels in the genitals.

❋ Testosterone cream, usually about $\frac{1}{2}$ gram per application, works wonders for many women when applied directly to the genital area before sexual activity.

5.
Sleep Disturbances—
Three Scenarios

Hygeia was an ancient Greek goddess of healing, and her eldest daughter was named Panacea. The word panacea means universal, or global, or affecting everything. If there is a true panacea for human health and well-being, it is a good night's sleep, every night. One of the most disturbing aspects of hormonal changes is their potential to continuously and maddeningly disrupt normal sleep cycles.

Normal sleeping comprises several aspects, including regularity of bedtime, a general sense of comfort in one's bed, a willingness to let go of solving problems for the day, and a series of cycling brain wave patterns. A good night's sleep has two or maybe three REM sleep cycles, and REM sleep is what we need to promote tissue regeneration and cellular healing. The first cycle is generally about four hours long. A brief waking after four hours is not necessarily deleterious as long as you can readily fall back to sleep. The next cycle will last up to three hours, and a final cycle, if available, will last about forty-five minutes to an hour.

The many hormonal changes that occur when you are approaching menopause can disturb a previously sound sleeper. Before discussing these changes specifically, here are a handful of general tips to help restore a good sleep pattern.

- Go to bed and get up at the same time every day.
- Make your sleep environment as comfortable as possible.
- Keep your bedroom as dark and as quiet as possible.
- Avoid caffeine stimulants—in chocolate, coffee, sodas, and tea—in the evening.

- Don't drink alcohol or smoke before going to bed.

- Get some exercise every day, but not in the evening hours.

- Don't nap in the daytime.

- Develop a sleep ritual—a nightly routine that eases you down from the day's activities.

- Use your bedroom for sleeping instead of working, worrying, or watching TV.

- If you can't sleep, try to simply rest deeply.

Establish a Bedtime Ritual

Try not to get agitated about not sleeping and don't watch the clock. When you are still and relaxed in bed, your metabolism slows down and you can get nearly as much benefit from this rest as you can if you were asleep. Understanding this will hopefully alleviate anxiety about not sleeping until you figure out what you need to do to actually fall asleep and stay asleep every night. Dr. Deepak Chopra has some good ideas about the sleep ritual. He writes that "the five senses are the gateways to the mind and body," and that by pacifying the five senses, the mind and body will become more relaxed and accessible to sleep. He suggests:

- **Sound.** Music with a slow rhythm and a deep pitch will help slow your metabolism. It stimulates the release of natural valium-type compounds in the body. The best time to listen to music is from 6 P.M. to 10 P.M.

- **Touch.** When touched gently, the skin releases soothing, relaxing chemicals. One simple way to achieve this is to massage the bottoms of your feet at bedtime with warm sesame oil. Sponge it off with a cool cloth after a few minutes.

- **Sight.** Your bedroom should be as visually pleasing as possible. An aquarium or a beautiful painting can be particularly restful. A warm, soothing color scheme promotes sleep.

- **Taste.** Have a glass of warm milk or a small handful of almonds at bedtime.

- **Smell.** The sense of smell directly influences the nervous system. The aromas of basil, clove, lavender, and orange have been shown to induce relaxation.

One way to combine all these ideas is to take a bath with a few drops of essential oil in the water, light a candle or two, have some soothing music going, and bring your snack or herbal tea into the bathroom with you. Although a hot bath is tempting, a neutral temperature bath (about body temperature, or 98 degrees Fahrenheit) is much more soothing. A hot bath that turns your skin pink is actually quite stimulating, as it enhances blood flow.

Herbal Sleep Aids

There is a wide array of herbal medicines that help summon Morpheus, the god of sleep.

- *Avena sativa* (oat straw). This is the familiar kitchen item frequently eaten as oatmeal. In fact, oats are one of the most universally used medicinal foods to soothe the nerves. You may want to eat your oats in the evening instead of at breakfast to ensure a restful sleep, but don't eat anything too close to bedtime. In general, no food should be taken closer than two hours before bedtime so your digestive workings don't keep you awake. Oats may also be used as a soothing bath: put a handful in an old sock and let the bath water run through the sock so the water becomes slightly slippery. Bathe in this gentle brew to allow the mildly sedative qualities to seep in through your skin. You can also take oats in a tincture form, beginning after dinner and taking frequent doses at short intervals. You should find tincture of avena at most health food stores.

- *Humulus lupulus* (hops, a popular flavoring for beer) can allay irritation or anxiety, thus promoting sleep. This isn't necessarily an endorsement for beer drinking. A better approach would be to rest your head at night on a pillow filled with dried hops leaves.

- *Lavendula officinalis* (lavender flower) works primarily through the sense of smell. It is extremely soothing to simply sniff a small opened bottle of the volatile oil made from these redolent blossoms. Many health food stores carry some brand of lavender oil. Keep it next to your bed or add a few drops to the bath water before retiring.

- *Leonorus cardiaca* (motherwort) is particularly useful for lack of sleep due to heart problems, including a broken heart. This herb is traditionally known to gladden the heart.

- *Matricaria recucita* (German chamomile, or any chamomile species) is helpful for sleep disturbed by anxiety or irritability. This herb is especially good for children. Take note: if you are using chamomile in a tea (infusion) form, don't let it steep more than three to five minutes. A strong chamomile tea can actually be mildly stimulating.

- *Melissa officinalis* (lemon balm) is a tasty plant that can soothe a nervous heart or a nervous stomach and therefore help with insomnia.

- *Passiflora incarnata* (passionflower) is a relaxing nervine, indicated for sleep disturbed by mental worries or anxiety, and for insomnia caused by fear.

- *Piscidia erythrina* (Jamaican dogwood) is a plant originally used to stun fish in ponds to make them easier to catch. It is great as a gentle pain reliever and for general nervousness, but can be toxic in high doses.

- *Scutellaria lateriflora* (skullcap) is another sweet-tasting herb to help alleviate nightmares or restless sleep. This herb combines well with passionflower and also helps to soothe intestinal cramps.

- *Valerian spp.* (valerian) has an active ingredient similar to the chemical forming the basis of many benzodiazepines, such as Valium. It can both relax and stimulate the central nervous system but don't use this botanical medicine in high doses for more than three weeks at a time. It combines well with hops.

There are also numerous effective Chinese medicinal herbs to choose from, including coptis, polygala, rhemannia, and schizandra. A lovely Western mixture for an herbal night pillow is hops leaves, lavender flowers, oregano, thyme, and valerian root. If there is an herbalist in your area, you can ask them to make this up for you, or ask a nutritionally oriented doctor for a referral to an herbal supply company. A mugwort leaf pillow is said to make for happy dreams.

Another great way to take sleep-inducing plants is in the form of a cup of tea before bed. An excellent sample sedative mixture contains hops leaves, lemon balm leaves, and valerian root in equal parts. Use one to two teaspoons of the herb to one cup of boiling water. Infuse for at least fifteen minutes and drink one cup before retiring. Use on a regular basis. Another sedative tea formula contains: 2 parts angelica root, 2 parts hops leaves, 3 parts lemon balm leaf, 1 part rosemary leaf, 1 part yarrow flowers. Follow above directions for steeping.

How Food Affects Sleep

Your dietary choices can also affect the quality of your sleep over time. Tryptophan is an amino acid (from the breakdown of protein) that is a precursor to the sleep neurotransmitter serotonin. It is naturally present in low levels in bananas, dairy products, eggs, fish, pineapples, turkey, walnuts, and whole wheat. You can also supplement with tryptophan, or the concentrated and more widely available form of tryptophan, 5-HTP (5-hydroxy tryptophan), 50–250 mg at bedtime. Tryptophan absorption is enhanced by a small carbohydrate snack and the concomitant use of vitamins B_3, B_6, and C (but these vitamins don't need to be taken at bedtime). Foods to avoid, especially in the afternoon and evening because they are stimulants, include alcohol, caffeine, fatty foods, fried foods, hot sauces, meat, rich, salty, or sweet foods, spicy foods, and sugar.

Melatonin

Low-dose melatonin is another therapeutic possibility for reestablishing good sleep patterns. I advocate using 0.5 mg at bedtime, which is just slightly more than average circulating levels in humans with adequate melatonin production. Melatonin became an overnight sensation after it was featured on the cover of *Newsweek* in August 1995. It remains controversial, although according to some reports melatonin has become more widely used to help combat the insomnia that plagues more than 6 million Americans. I am increasingly impressed with the safety and efficacy of this naturally occurring hormone when it is used judiciously and in small doses. Melatonin levels have been shown to decline dramatically and predictably with age, although this finding has been disputed.

Melatonin is the primary secretion of the pineal gland, a pine-nut sized gland set deep in the brain behind the third-eye area (between and slightly above the eyebrows). The pineal gland is connected both to the retina at the back of the eyes, and to the pituitary and hypothalamus, the master endocrine glands. Melatonin secretion kicks in as the sun goes down and the intensity of light through the eyes onto the retina begins to fade, and it is thought to be a major regulator of sleep. In biochemical terms melatonin is directly downstream from tryptophan, which converts to 5-HTP, which becomes serotonin, and then melatonin. So melatonin's lineage is from the sleep-inducing, feel-good hormones, tryptophan and serotonin.

The relationship of melatonin to other endocrine secretions has to do with the ebb and flow of hormonal release into the bloodstream throughout the day. Sometimes this daily rhythm is referred to as circadian rhythm, circadian meaning "about a day," from the Latin *circa* and *dia*. The evolution of life forms on this planet is intrinsically linked with the rising and setting of the sun, and most life forms today require both periods of light and periods of dark to thrive. In animals with a seasonal breeding pattern, changing levels of melatonin (as the days grow longer in the spring) trigger changes in the secretion of reproductive hormones. Melatonin has been shown to reduce testosterone and prolactin levels, and is thought to increase estrogen levels. It is known that melatonin interacts with other hormones, but the ramification of all the interactions remains to be fully understood. Recent research into melatonin as a potent antioxidant has prompted leading cancer treatment centers to incorporate a relatively high dose (20 mg) of melatonin both in treating various (mostly hormonal) cancers and in combating the potentially devastating side effects of conventional cancer treatment, namely radiation and chemotherapy.

The controversy around melatonin as a sleep-inducing agent revolves around whether supplementation is useful in people who have what is considered to be adequate innate melatonin levels. Several studies imply that the sleep-promoting effects of melatonin are only apparent if melatonin levels are low. Since we do know that light inhibits melatonin synthesis, it makes sense that melatonin may be less effective in the winter months. Remember to avoid turning on the light if you get up to use the bathroom at night, because light will inhibit melatonin secretion.

Few problematic side effects have been attributed to melatonin use, but I recommend avoiding using melatonin if you are pregnant or attempting to become pregnant since it has been shown to increase miscarriage rates in experimental lab rats.

Getting to Sleep and Staying Asleep

Another way to analyze sleep disturbances is to ask yourself whether the problem is getting to sleep or staying asleep. If your problem is getting to sleep, consider melatonin (0.5 mg at bedtime) or a tincture, or tea, of some of the herbs mentioned above. A soothing bedtime routine, including a tepid bath with epsom salts (magnesium sulfate, my favorite muscle relaxant, which absorbs nicely through the skin) and a few drops of lavender oil should prove helpful. If the problem is staying asleep, one cause may be nighttime hypoglycemia. Your blood sugar may dip down low enough during the night to cause wakefulness. If this occurs, try a light bedtime snack, such as half a banana or a small handful of almonds. You might also take notice of the time of night you wake and note if it is usually the same time. Traditional Chinese medicine (TCM) has recognized a circadian pattern of organ function, for example the liver meridian is active from 1 A.M.–3 A.M. and the lung meridian from 3 A.M.–5 A.M. If you regularly wake up at a certain time of night, a licensed acupuncturist in your community will be able to help you balance your energy to promote smooth flowing of the vital force (the Chinese call it *Qi*, pronounced *chee,* which literally means steaming rice) within your energy channels (meridians). Health, from the perspective of TCM, is both a smooth flow of the Qi and a balanced level of Qi in each of the fourteen major meridians.

Is There a Hormone Connection?

Good luck trying to figure out the relationship of sex hormones to sleep patterns. High estrogen and low estrogen, high progesterone and low progesterone are all affiliated with disrupted sleep. Determining which of your hormones is out of balance cannot be done from the symptom of sleep disturbance alone. You'll need to look at the whole picture with a healthcare provider familiar with signs and symptoms of hormonal changes. (Chapter 11 contains a table listing the effects of high and low levels of estrogen or progesterone.) I recommend first trying nonhormonal approaches to restoring good sleep. As Hippocrates reputedly said, "Let food be thy medicine, and medicine thy food." Benjamin Franklin wrote, "If illness can be cured by diet, it should not be cured any other way." If you feel you need hormonal measures to restore sleep, as a starting point you could try progesterone supplementation during the second half of your cycle if you are still menstruating, and bioidentical estrogen if you are no longer bleeding.

Maybe the main reason you are not sleeping well at night is hot flashes, or even more disturbing, episodes of drenching night sweats. The next chapter contains natural remedies for these problems.

Treatment Summary

❋ Keep regular hours and try to eat your meals at similar times each day. It is especially important is to eat dinner well before bedtime because going to bed with a full stomach is not restful. Try to go to bed and wake up at similar times each day, including weekend days.

❋ Avoid stimulants if you are a light sleeper. Coffee is notorious for disrupting sound sleep, even if it is only ingested in the morning.

❋ There is a wide array of wonderful, safe, readily available herbal nervines—plant medicines that soothe the central nervous system—and most of them can be taken in tea form. (Refer to this chapter's list of herbal remedies that restore optimal sleep.)

❋ A light carbohydrate snack at bedtime (such as half a banana or a piece of toast with honey) with some protein (such as nuts or a bite of fish) will not only prevent your blood sugar from dropping too low during the night, but will also promote levels of a sleep-inducing protein in the blood: tryptophan. This naturally occurring protein is the precursor to serotonin, the feel-good brain chemical that makes Prozac (and other selective serotonin reuptake inhibitors) work.

❋ My personal favorite sleep aid is melatonin. I use only low doses (only 0.5 mg at bedtime). The new research on melatonin keeps making it look better. It is also a potent antioxidant and is now being used in many cancer treatments.

6.

Hot Flashes and Night Sweats— When Will This Stop?

If I had to choose one symptom of menopause and perimenopause that drives women the craziest, it definitely would be hot flashes. This often brings women to the doctor's office, because they just can't stand the embarrassment and uncertainty of extreme temperature surges and drenching sweats. Up to 65 percent of perimenopausal women experience this annoying and inconsistent symptom, and most women who have stopped bleeding will experience hot flashes during the first two years after the onset of menopause.

Hot flashes vary dramatically in intensity and frequency. Some women mostly have hot flashes at night, when they can produce night sweats. Some women have them every hour on the hour throughout the day and have to change their clothes several times. Some women simply get a little hot under the collar from time to time for a few years. The average duration of a hot flash is three and a half minutes, but they can be as quick as five seconds and as prolonged as an hour. Although many women experience hot flashes all over their bodies, most hot flashes are felt primarily in the face and chest area, sometimes in the breast area, and occasionally in the hands and feet. Hot flashes may be accompanied by the sensation of your heart racing, or you may break out in a sweat. There is no predictable, typical pattern. Some women get hot flashes while their menses are still regular. Some women only begin to get hot flashes when their periods are starting to become irregular, and then only during non-bleeding days. Some women don't start to get hot flashes until several years after their menses have stopped, and once in a while there is a woman who gets no hot flashes at all.

Temperature Swings

The medical term for the hot flash is vasomotor instability. I mention this because it may be interesting for you to know exactly what is happening in a hot flash. Vasomotor refers to the ability of a blood vessel to expand and contract, which is how the nervous system directs blood more intensively to the area of the body that needs it. For example, after eating a meal, the digestive system needs more blood, so blood is directed to the stomach and intestines. When exercising, the major muscles used for physical movement as well as the lungs and heart need more blood, so blood is shunted away from the digestive organs and into the legs and cardiovascular system. What is happening in a hot flash is a hormonally driven rise in temperature, almost like a mini-fever. The body immediately tries to cool off by moving the blood toward the surface of the body. This is why hot flashes can be brought on by hot weather, spicy foods, and warm drinks, all of which heat up the body. Other potential triggers are alcohol, caffeine, chocolate, stress, and very salty foods.

The Ovaries and the Brain Are Not in Sync

The way hormones induce hot flashes is not fully understood, but it goes something like this: As hormone levels decrease (first progesterone, then estrogen), the brain gets the message that the ovaries need more of a push to secrete more of these hormones. So the ovaries, which are actually trying to retire at this point, gather up their remaining strength and finally respond to the brain by releasing hormones in a surge similar to what happens at ovulation in a regularly menstruating woman. One of the ways to determine when ovulation occurs, in fact, is to check your temperature every morning. There is almost always a slight temperature rise right at ovulation, which indicates that the ovaries have responded to the brain by releasing more hormones. What goes up, must come down, so after the temporary rise in hormones (either at ovulation, or in the perimenopausal woman, preceding a hot flash), there is an equally sudden drop in hormone levels, which is what causes the hot flash symptom through the vasomotor action in the blood vessels. I'm going into this explanation to let you know that, besides hormone treatment, an effective approach to reducing the intensity and frequency of hot flashes is to stabilize the blood vessels' response to temperature fluctuations.

Plant Antihistamines Stabilize Blood Vessels

Bioflavonoids will be extensively discussed in Chapter 12, but as a brief introduction, let's start with the word itself. *Bio* means coming from nature, and *flavonoid* means yellow-colored. Bioflavonoids are found in many plants, but especially in colorful fruits and vegetables. I like to think of bioflavonoids as natural antihistamines, because they reduce the rush of blood to areas of the body, such as the eyes, nose, and throat, which occurs when exposed to allergens. (Many of you are familiar with over-the-counter antihistamines, such as Benadryl or Contact.) Histamine is a substance released from certain blood cells, mostly the platelets, which causes more fluid and blood to rush to the area of the body besieged by allergens. The allergens may be environmental, such as dander, dust, or pollen, or they may be food-based. Some of the most allergy inducing foods are corn (especially corn syrup), dairy products, nuts (especially peanuts), shellfish, soy, and wheat. Some people are sensitive to more unusual food allergens, such as citrus fruits, garlic, gluten-containing grains, and meats. If you suspect you have allergies, work with a doctor familiar with testing and treating them. Histamine responses to allergens can definitely make hot flashes worse. My favorite bioflavonoid for treating hot flashes and allergies (both of which involve histamine dumping) is quercetin, derived from the yellow-orange pigment in plants. You may need a fair amount of quercetin to get good results. I recommend 1,000 mg several times daily, taken with food, as all supplements should be, to enhance absorption.

Many plant medicines have been used to help control hot flashes. They work as natural antihistamines, or to block estrogen surges, or both. One naturopathic study found good effect from the following formulation:

- 2 parts *Angelica sinensis* (dong quai root), which increases progesterone secretion;

- 2 parts *Arctium lappa* (burdock root), which contains plant estrogens;

- 1 part *Dioscorea barbasco* (Mexican wild yam root), which is considered to be a phytoestrogen (meaning it works like soy to block excess estrogen);

- 2 parts *Glycyrrhiza glabra* (licorice root), which contains bioflavonoids and inhibits excess estrogen activity;

- 1 part *Leonorus cardiaca* (motherwort), which is traditionally used as a uterine tonic to support the reproductive system.

Sage

My favorite plant medicine for hot flashes is garden-variety sage (*Salvia offici-*

nalis). Although there is very little research on common sage the Chinese medicinal plant *Salvia miltiorrhiza* (dan shen), a relative, has been shown to increase estrogen levels in lab rats. When women are having hot flashes while still menstruating, the problem is probably excess estrogen and sage may not work as well. If you are no longer menstruating, sage may work well for you. I recommend several cups of cooled sage tea daily. My favorite brand is Female Sage from Traditional Medicinals. This company uses organically grown plants in their teas whenever possible. They also use a nontoxic sealant for the tea bags. Whenever you use herbal medicine, sniff the exposed herb. It should smell lively. Don't bother with a plant-based supplement that has no taste or smell.

Black Cohosh

If you are still menstruating, you may find the herbal medicine black cohosh (*Cimicifuga racemosa*) more effective than sage. Standardized black cohosh is perhaps the most researched of all the plant medicines for treating symptoms of perimenopause. Standardized black cohosh has been widely marketed as Remifemin to help control hot flashes. This medicine, which came out of Germany, was so popular that it was bought out in 2001 by the pharmaceutical giant Glaxo, which is now selling it at five times the original price. Much more affordable and as effective is the original product now called "AM/PM" sold under the Integrative Therapeutics brand. However, any standardized black cohosh from a reputable supplement company should give good relief from intense and frequent hot flashes. I recommend starting with 20 mg in the morning and 20 mg at bedtime. You can safely increase the dose to 400 mg daily, in 2 doses of 200 mg each. If you aren't helped by 400 mg daily, black cohosh will probably not do the trick for you. If higher doses do help, reduce the dose to the lowest effective amount when possible. Although there is no evidence suggesting that black cohosh could increase the risk of hormonally driven cancers (breast, uterus, womb), the theoretical possibility exists.

The Joy of Soy

Another well-documented phytoestrogen is soy. Apparently, Japanese women have no word for hot flash. However, Japanese-Americans who no longer eat a traditional Japanese diet high in soy products and sea vegetables get hot flashes the way any other American woman might. So, it's not genetics but the diet that seems to make the difference in Japanese women. You may need

40–60 grams of soy protein daily to control hot flashes. Most soy products, including soy protein powders, will list the amount of soy protein per serving size. Besides protein powders, you may enjoy stirring miso paste into warm water to make a nutritive broth, or munching on a handful of dry roasted soy nuts, or cubing a block of tofu to add to a stir-fry instead of meat or fish. Tofu comes in different textures and is almost tasteless on its own. Experiment with your favorite blends of spices to season the tofu. Silken tofu is the softest and best for blending; you can use it to make shakes with added fruit juice or berries. Firm tofu can be put into soups, curries, or pasta dishes, as well as stir-fries.

Another benefit of soy is that is it high in calcium, so it can help protect bones. On the downside, soy has been reported to inhibit thyroid function, so it is a good idea to eat it in combination with foods containing thyroid-enhancing iodine. Foods such as fish and sea vegetables are good choices because they are naturally high in iodine. Even though soy has estrogenlike properties, it seems to protect against breast and uterine cancer because, as previously stated, it blocks estrogen receptors from absorbing excess estrogen.

Always use organic soy products; otherwise, you will be eating GMO food—that is, food that has been genetically modified.

Progesterone

If you are still menstruating, progesterone derived from plants may be the best choice for you to offset estrogen dominance. Avoid the chemical progestins, which are affiliated with breast and uterine cancer. Start with 100 mg daily, in lozenge or cream form, during the second half of your menstrual cycle. If your periods are irregular, take the progesterone two weeks on, two weeks off. If you are no longer menstruating, that means not only is the progesterone gone, but the estrogen is starting to wane also. Progesterone is not particularly useful in a nonmenstruating woman (other than to protect the uterus against cancer when taking estrogen replacement therapy). Estrogen will fairly reliably arrest hot flashes in a menopausal woman. I strongly recommend using only plant-based estrogens that are manipulated in the laboratory to be identical to human estrogen. (See Chapter 11 on Bioidentical Hormones.)

Dress in Layers

You have probably already figured out how to dress in layers to accommodate unpredictable hot flashes. You should also avoid synthetic fabrics, turtlenecks, and any clothing that is too complicated to take off quickly. It may also help to think of hot flashes as power surges. Try to remember that hot flashes are a sign of passing through to a stage in life that represents greater maturity, personal power, and wisdom. At least you can try to keep these ideas in mind between power surges. If all the above is not working well enough for you, there is always the hormone option.

Treatment Summary

❋ Black cohosh is a plant medicine with a long history of being a uterine and ovarian tonic. Take 40 mg daily: 20 mg in the morning and 20 mg at bedtime. Black cohosh works even better if you also supplement with 800 IU of vitamin E daily. Black cohosh contains plant estrogens.

❋ Many other plant medicines (which do not have compounds that mimic hormones) can help with perimenopausal hot flashes. A few of my favorites are angelica (dong quai root), burdock root, red clover, and sage. These can be taken in capsule, alcohol extraction, or tea form. Check with your local health food store.

❋ Eat a daily serving of soy-based foods, such as one-quarter block of tofu, or one tablespoon miso (fermented soybean paste) or a half cup of roasted soy nuts. Soy is also a plant estrogen, but unlike human or horse estrogen it reduces the risk of breast and uterine cancer.

❋ Natural hormones mean progesterone (if you are still having periods) or estrogen plus progesterone from plant sources, which are converted in a laboratory to hormones that are *identical* to human progesterone and estrogens. Avoid hormones that are extracted from the urine of pregnant animals (usually mares). Work with a holistically oriented doctor to obtain the correct prescription.

❋ Dress in layers and avoid getting overheated. This also means minimizing alcohol, hot beverages, and spicy foods.

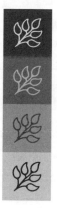

7.

Getting Shorter?
You Don't Have To

Osteoporosis has reached epidemic proportions in the United States. Men are not exempt. Check your height every year and talk to your doctor if you have lost more than one inch. Osteoporosis is preventable. It's much harder to reverse.

Healthy Bones Are Flexible

One of the effects of waning hormones is a reduction in bone density. The result of this, osteoporosis, is responsible for more than 1 million hospitalizations because of fractures every year in the United States. Estrogen helps the bone-building cells to multiply and maintain optimal bone density for strength and flexibility. But bones need more than estrogen to stay strong. They also need many different minerals, including calcium, moving in and out from blood to bone and back to blood. What many people don't know about bones is that they are not actually solid or rigid. They are quite porous, and minerals constantly keep flowing off and onto the bone. Solid materials, such as a wooden table, only *appear* solid because the molecules are so close together and are moving around so quickly you can't easily penetrate between them. The same is true with bone. It *appears* solid, but the ions flow on and off in a highly dynamic way, which actually gives bounce to the bone and makes it stronger and more flexible.

You may have heard about the importance of weight-bearing exercise for keeping bones strong. When people are confined to hospital beds, for even a short time, they quickly lose bone mass because of the lack of pressure, or weight-bearing, on the long bones of their bodies. In fact, the latest hospital beds have a way to press people's head and feet toward each other for 10 minutes twice a day to put pressure on the long bones, somewhat like a reverse rack. This pressure, or weight-bearing, slightly bends the flexible long bones, making the bones curve. Positively charged minerals (such as calcium and magnesium) gather on one side of the curve and negatively charged minerals (such as chloride) gather on the other side. The positive charge on one side of the bone and the negative charge on the other side create an electrical current, much like a battery. Bones are lively because they are actually electric. But they only stay charged and lively when they are slightly curved. That is why weight-bearing exercise to keep the bones slightly curved is so important for bone strength.

You Need More Than Calcium

Many women are taking extra calcium to keep their bones strong, but beware: calcium alone does not make for strong bones. Further, dairy products are not an optimal way to obtain calcium, mainly because humans are not designed to digest cow's milk. Even adult cows don't drink cow's milk. Another problem with cow's milk is that, besides calcium, it generally comes with plenty of cholesterol and antibiotics. The countries with the highest consumption of dairy products (United States, Finland, Sweden, and England) also happen to be the same four countries with the highest incidence of osteoporosis. Coincidence? Probably not. On average, African-Americans consume more than 1,000 mg of calcium daily, mostly from dairy sources, and have a nine times greater incidence of hip fracture than black South Africans, who consume under 200 mg of calcium daily from sources other than dairy. Bone structure is much more complex than calcium alone. Supplementing with calcium alone may actually make the bones brittle and *more* susceptible to fracture. This does not mean calcium is bad. On the contrary, calcium is the most abundant mineral in the body as the main element in the skeleton and teeth. About 2 percent of the total body weight is from calcium. The circulating calcium (floating around in the blood) is tightly controlled. We pull calcium from the bones if we need more in the blood to trigger many bodily functions, such as muscle contractions to keep the heart pumping.

Calcium carbonate is a reasonably good, and inexpensive, form for supplementing calcium, but if you have trouble absorbing calcium, as many do, calcium citrate is the form most likely to be well-absorbed by the body. Adolescent girls should ingest 1,300–1,500 mg of calcium daily, and this can drop to 1,000 mg daily after age twenty. In the perimenopausal years, depending on how much calcium you get from your diet, you may want to increase the calcium to 1,300–1,500 mg daily again until several years beyond menopause. But take calcium with vitamin D and with other minerals in a multimineral supplement that includes boron (up to 3 mg), magnesium, and ideally also strontium.

Bone-Building Basics

The basics for good bone building include not only calcium but also vitamin D, vitamin K, magnesium, manganese, folic acid, boron, strontium, silicon, vitamin B_6, zinc, copper, and vitamin C. Any bone-building supplement would ideally feature these listed nutrients. Some recent research suggests that strontium may be the most important bone nutrient after calcium. Here's a brief review of why these nutrients are important.

- **Vitamin D,** required for the absorption of calcium in the intestine, is not actually a vitamin at all: it's more like a hormone. Vitamin D deficiencies are surprisingly common, particularly in older women, and especially in the winter. And those living above 40 degrees north of the equator (Denver, Indianapolis, Philadelphia, Reno) will run out of vitamin D stores despite getting outside daily. Vitamin D deficiency is associated not only with osteoporosis but also with higher rates of cancer of the breast, colon, ovary, prostate, and rectum. The daily minimum requirement for those over age fifty is 400 IU, and those over age seventy need 600 IU. If you are under fifty years old and get outside regularly, 200 IU daily will be enough.

- **Vitamin K** is required for the formation of osteocalcin, a protein that attracts calcium onto the bone structure.

- **Magnesium** activates the formation of new calcium crystals, which allows the calcium to be incorporated into the bone structure. In addition, magnesium is critical to many cellular functions because it can activate enzymes that work within the cells. This work includes cellular replication, energy production, and protein formation. About 60 percent of the body's magnesium is found in bone, 26 percent in muscle (it is a potent muscle relaxant) and the rest in the soft tissue and body fluids. The tissues with the highest concentration of magnesium are the brain, heart, kidneys, and liver—in other words, highly active organs. Magnesium is essential to these critical organs, and the typical American diet is low in magnesium. I recommend 400 mg daily.

- **Manganese** is also required for bone minerals to acquire the crystalline form which allows them to become part of our bone structure. Women with osteoporosis typically have only 25 percent of the amount of manganese as those with healthy bones.

- **Folic acid** prevents the buildup of a protein residue called homocysteine, which leads not only to bone loss, but also to heart disease. Drinking alcohol, smoking tobacco, and using oral contraceptives all cause folic acid deficiency.

- **Boron** is a trace mineral that helps estrogen be more effective in maintaining strong bones and helps make calcium intake more efficient.

- **Strontium** is a natural component of healthy bones and teeth. Natural strontium is not radioactive. Researcher Jonathan Wright, M.D., feels strontium is the most important bone builder after calcium. He and Alan Gaby, M.D., have formulated a bone-building supplement that I have used in my practice for more than ten years.

- **Silicon** helps to interconnect the various mineral components of bone.

- **Vitamin B$_6$,** like folic acid, prevents homocysteine buildup, and like silicon, helps link together the diverse components of bone.

- **Zinc** is an essential trace mineral for bone formation, and enhances vitamin D activity.

- **Copper** is thought to help with bone structure.

- **Vitamin C** deficiency results not only in scurvy (once common in sailors, now rare) but also in osteoporosis.

My favorite bone-building supplement is OsteoPrime by PhytoPharmica. It was formulated by two leading nutritionally oriented physician-researchers and should be available in health food stores or progressive pharmacies throughout the country. Beyond supplementation, your dietary choices are of paramount importance in maintaining bone density and preventing unnecessary bone loss.

Sodas Destroy Bone

A diet with lots of processed foods and a high sugar content is likely to be deficient in the bone nutrients discussed above. If you fill up on sugary, junk-food snacks, you won't eat mineral-rich foods like dark, leafy greens (best steamed), other vegetables, or healthful fruits. Everyone should have at least one and a half cups of fresh or steamed vegetables daily, plus at least one piece of whole fruit. A high-protein diet, such as daily meat, tends to make our intestinal tract more acid. The blood needs to be slightly alkaline (the opposite of acid) and we would quickly die if our blood became too acidic, meaning that when we eat acid-forming foods (like animal protein, grains, or sugar), our bodies need to neutralize the acid with alkaline minerals. Those alkaline minerals come from the bones. So, if we make a habit of eating mostly acid-forming foods, we eventually strip alkaline minerals off the bones.

Among the very worst foods for bones, especially horrible for teenage girls growing their adult bones, are carbonated soft drinks—sodas. Not only does each soda contain an incredible amount of sugar—twelve tablespoons per can—but the fizz is created by adding phosphoric acid to the brew. This very acidic liquid strongly pulls the alkaline minerals (mostly calcium and magnesium) out of the bone and will eventually cause irreversible bone loss. I consider it criminal to allow these carbonated soft drinks to be sold in public schools.

Stay Balanced

We talked about how many people, mostly women, go to the hospital each year with broken bones, and how estrogen, minerals, weight-bearing exercise, and a diet rich in fruits and vegetables can reduce this problem. Another consideration in the bone-health equation is maintaining good balance. Think about it. Even if your bones have become somewhat more fragile with age, if you don't fall, you won't break a bone. The most common bones that fracture in older women with weakened bones are the hip, the wrist, and parts of the spine. It is not uncommon for an elderly woman to go to the hospital with a broken hip, catch pneumonia in the hospital, and die. You don't have to become one of those little old ladies. Eat your vegetables. Stay active. Practice balance exercises.

One of the best ways to maintain good balance is the stretching technique known as yoga. Yoga means union in Sanskrit, an ancient East Indian language, and the practice of yoga will help you attain union of body, mind, and spirit. The root of the word yoga is the same word as yoke, as in yoking oxen together in the field to draw the plow. Many yoga poses are based on excellent posture, with an emphasis on flexibility of the spine. Most of us only use our spines to bend forward, but the spine is perfectly capable of bending sideways and backward as well. Unless we practice those motions the spine will slowly become rigid and stiff. Yoga helps us keep our spines flexible and maintain excellent posture.

The practice of yoga also teaches us how to balance. Quite a few yoga poses, such as the tree pose, involve standing on one leg. If you can balance on one foot for sixty seconds or more you probably have good balance and will be much less likely to fall and break a bone. Balance is an ability that declines with age without practice. Try to balance on one foot, then the other foot, for at least one minute every day. Try it with your eyes closed to make this exercise more challenging. Practice makes perfect. If you like the feeling of being more balanced and flexible, you may want to explore the yoga community in your area. Aim for two to three yoga sessions weekly. Yogis say that you are as young as your spine is flexible, and yoga is a wonderful way to stay flexible in body, mind, and spirit. It will also greatly reduce your chances of broken bones later in life.

Measuring Bone Density

How can you determine your bone density? You need to get a specialized x-ray called a DEXA (which stands for dual x-ray absorptiometry) to accurately measure the strength of the bone at the most vulnerable points of the body (lower spinal vertebrae, wrist, and where the top of the leg connects to the hip). Most communities greater than 20,000 people will have a medical or osteopathic doctor or a chiropractor who provides this service. The test is fairly expensive, usually $200 and up. This special x-ray machine reads your bone at two or three sites, and then the computer program built into the machine figures out your "T" score. A T score in the positive range (above zero) is excellent. A minus number (down to minus 2) means bone loss compared to other women your age, which is called osteopenia. Minus 2.5 or lower signifies osteoporosis, which literally mean "holes in the bones."

The DEXA will give you a score of your current bone density, but it won't tell you if you are losing bone, or whether your bone loss occurred a while back and is now stable. It does not help you determine what your bone density score will be next year. A better test to screen for ongoing bone loss is a urine test that measures byproducts of bone breakdown. Most doctors offering this test have patients take it home because you need to collect your first morning urine after you wake up to send to the lab. This test is not as expensive (usually about $65), and it lets you know if you are currently losing bone. If possible, arrange to have both tests done together.

Once a DEXA scan has established that the bone density of my premenopausal patient is good, I can keep track of that woman's bone health with the urine test once or twice a year until she is three to five years past menopause. As long as she is not actively losing bone, I don't have to worry about her bone density dipping toward osteoporosis. If she does start losing bone, I can implement treatment right away and then monitor the effectiveness of the treatment through continued urine tests and DEXA scans.

Another very simple way to keep track of possible bone loss is through measurement of height. Measure your height every year starting at age thirty-five, especially if you have family members with osteoporosis. If you lose more than half an inch from one year to the next, and you are under age fifty, consider getting further evaluation to confirm the possibility of bone loss. Another late sign of osteoporosis is loose teeth. That implies bone loss in the jaw, and in every other bone, as well. Remember that it is much easier to prevent osteoporosis than to treat it.

Bones and Hormones

Now, let's discuss the relationship between hormones and bones. There are three main types of estrogen: E1, E2, and E3. Most of the research relating to bone density has shown that the active estrogen is E2 (also known as estradiol). The optimal blood level of estradiol to maintain strong bones is 50–150 units. Your estradiol level can be determined through a blood test available at any doctor's office. I always use estrogen (even the bioidentical natural variety of the hormone) as a last resort if a patient has a low level of estradiol, because of the potential for the unwanted side effects of estrogen supplementation, such as breast cancer (relatively rare) and more commonly, blood clots. See Chapter 11 for more on the topic of bioidentical hormones.

Unless your uterus has been surgically removed, progesterone must be taken along with estrogen to prevent uterine cancer because estrogen alone increases the risk of uterine cancer. Progesterone is not useful in maintaining bone density, contrary to some widely published material, but it does offset the risk of uterine cancer. Some studies suggest that estrogen and progesterone together can have a positive synergistic effect on bone, but no good studies exist to support the idea that progesterone alone strengthens bones. I do not intend to discredit progesterone, however. On the contrary, progesterone (not the synthetic progestin, such as the drug Provera) can be extremely helpful in treating many premenopausal problems such as breast tenderness, hair loss, hot flashes, low libido, menstrual irregularity, mood swings, night sweats, vaginal dryness, and others. However, I want to emphatically make the point that progesterone alone is a poor choice if your main concern is bone loss.

Review your risk for bone loss with a trusted healthcare provider and have the appropriate testing to analyze your bone density. The more bone loss you have already experienced, the more aggressively you may need to be treated and monitored to prevent osteoporosis. Your chances of having rapid bone loss at menopause increase if you don't exercise, or if you eat meat regularly, have female relatives with osteoporosis, have never had children, smoke, take thyroid medications, or use prescription (steroidal) anti-inflammatories. Osteoporosis is a preventable disease, and worth preventing, since it can compromise your health and comfort in your older years.

Ipriflavone, Natural Bone Builder

An alternative to estrogen for stimulating bone growth is a synthetic isoflavone called ipriflavone. Isoflavones are a class of phytoestrogens found primarily in legumes (soy, for example) that are thought to have estrogenlike qualities, such as increasing bone density. Ipriflavone, at 600 mg daily, has been shown in numerous studies to prevent the breakdown of existing bone as well as increasing the formation of new bone. A few studies have drawn a correlation between reduced white blood cell counts and ipriflavone supplementation. Overall however, ipriflavone is much safer than estrogen, and might be a good choice before resorting to estrogen to improve your bone density.

Building Bone with Diet

Keep this in mind: what you put into your mouth will have a greater impact on your health than all of your other activities combined. Your body is made out of what you just ate. A bunch of steamed leafy greens, one and a half cups of cooked broccoli, half a cup of fortified tofu, and half a cup of sesame seeds not only contain *more* absorbable calcium than a cup of milk, but also less fat, no hormone or antibiotic residue, and many other minerals and vitamins that support overall health, including bone health. Finally, probably the most important nutritional advice I can give you for preventing bone loss is to stop drinking carbonated sodas, now and forever.

Treatment Summary

❀ Weight-bearing exercise is critical for bone health. Jumping rope is the very best, and jogging and weightlifting are also good. If you aren't ready for those activities, yoga will help strengthen *and* stretch, a winning combination. Aim for two to three sessions weekly of yoga, or running and weightlifting, or ideally all three activities.

❀ Take a multimineral supplement—not just calcium. Aim for minerals in food—think dark leafy vegetables—plus another 1,000 mg of supplemental calcium and magnesium.

❀ Vitamin D is the liquid sunshine that helps bones absorb minerals: Take 400 IU daily. My favorite form of vitamin D is cod liver oil. Carlson Laboratories makes a good lemon-lime flavored variety even my six year old loves.

❀ Carbonated soft drinks strip minerals from bones. Avoid them.

❀ Use estrogen as a last resort. There are several types of estrogen, but E2 has been definitively proven to increase bone mass. Choose bioidentical estrogen, which must be coupled with progesterone if you have a uterus. Your E2 (estradiol) blood levels should be at least 50 to maintain bone density. Ask your healthcare professional to help you get this checked. If estradiol in your blood is lower than 50 and your bone density scan (DEXA) shows bone loss, you may need to take estrogen for a few years to halt the loss, which can be rapid at the beginning of menopause.

8.

Foggy Thinking— I Can't Find My Keys . . . Again

oggy thinking means you feel as though your thoughts are coming through a thick fog. You can't remember conversations or events that transpired recently. Sometimes it is difficult to sort out whether or not foggy thinking is actually depression. Usually, however, it's clear to you that you're not depressed, except about the fact that you can't find your keys . . . again. Even though many people will joke about early Alzheimer's, this frightening disease is so common it is considered an epidemic in the United States today. Just because you tend to lose your keys doesn't mean you have Alzheimer's disease, of course, but on the other hand, do seek a professional evaluation of your mental and physical functioning if you are regularly getting confused about the normal tasks of daily life. Many cases of Alzheimer's disease can be prevented, or if genetically predestined, delayed.

Now Do I Need Hormones?

Both declining amounts of progesterone and declining amounts of estrogen can create foggy thinking. If you are still menstruating regularly, a course of natural progesterone may be a good choice for you. If you have stopped your period for at least six months, a course of the safest estrogen, E3 (estriol) might help with brain function. Progesterone can be found over the counter, unlike estrogen, but for either hormone I strongly urge you to work with a healthcare provider who is educated about all the options.

Drugs Drain Brains

Besides hormonal deficiencies, foggy thinking can also be caused by drug interactions, early cardiovascular disease, nutritional deficiencies, and toxic exposure. You will need a healthcare professional to help you sort this out. If you drink more than two ounces of alcohol daily, you may be so deficient in B vitamins that you can no longer think straight. A long history of birth control use is also known to deplete B vitamins. Vitamin B_{12} levels in the blood are significantly lower in patients with Alzheimer's disease, which may provide a clue. Zinc levels also tend to be very low in people with Alzheimer's and it may be that slightly low levels can cause foggy thinking. I'm not trying to say that foggy thinking leads to Alzheimer's. Rather, my point is that any form of mental decline is part of a continuum, from the small start of losing keys here and there to full-out not remembering your own name. By understanding the various factors that contribute to mental decline, we can help ourselves stay sharp and savvy well into old age. Doesn't that sound like more fun? It is certainly more fun for our friends and family.

One way to easily check zinc levels is the zinc tally test. Try to find some zinc lozenges that contain at least 30 mcg of zinc, or better yet, zinc in liquid form. Place a lozenge or a drop on your tongue. If it tastes quite metallic, that means your system has enough zinc to maintain a healthy immune system, which helps prevent free-radical damage to the brain. If the zinc is practically tasteless, that means you need zinc and should supplement with it, preferably in the zinc picolinate form. To be absorbed, zinc must be mixed with a secretion from the pancreas called picolinic acid. The pancreas is an important organ under the stomach; it produces digestive enzymes as well as bicarbonate of soda, which neutralizes the food in the stomach, and insulin, which helps control the levels of blood sugar. Pancreatic function declines with age, which is why most of us need help with optimum nutrient absorption as we get older. Look for zinc in the picolinate form and supplement with 30–50 mg daily if you need it.

Good Fats Keep the Brain Healthy

Another important dietary consideration, besides Vitamin B_{12} and the trace mineral zinc, is essential fatty acids. What I'm talking about here is good fat, the type that keeps your cells flexible and improves blood flow and electrical conductivity through the central nervous system. The central nervous system consists of the brain and spinal cord and is primarily made of fat. So, don't be insulted the next time someone calls you a fathead. The good fats are the ones that are linked together in wavy lines, without any help from hydrogen, which makes fats stiff and bereft of energy. Hydrogenated fats like margarine and Crisco have hydrogen forced onto them to preserve their shelf life, as they would otherwise become rancid fairly quickly. Remember, when choosing foods, aim for foods that would eventually become rotten, but eat them before they do. A food that would stay on the shelf, preserved indefinitely, is extremely suspect. Since fats are very prone to rot—go rancid—sniff your oils before eating them. Avoid oils that smell bad. Keeping them in dark-colored containers and away from heat will help make oils and fats last longer.

The most healing fat for the body, which we must eat because we can't produce it internally, is omega-3 (which refers to its biochemical structure). The best source of omega-3 fats is coldwater fish, such as salmon and tuna. The *only* plant source of omega-3 fats is flaxseed oil. Freshly ground flaxseeds rank in my top-five category of foods because of their health benefits and delicious taste.

Best Brain Foods

If I had to choose only five foods to eat for the rest of my life, that would be tough. But I'd probably choose fresh Alaskan salmon, ground-up flaxseeds, lightly pickled beets, ripe organic mangoes, steamed chard, and maybe even dark organic chocolate, for its antioxidant qualities and just because it is so tasty. Luckily, however, I don't have to choose because the choice of delicious and nutritious foods is astounding and provides a feast for the eyes and palate, as well as being the foundation of good health.

I recommend three tablespoons of freshly ground flaxseeds stirred into water or juice several times a week for optimal brain health. A major fringe benefit of consuming ground flaxseeds is regularity of bowel movements because the flax meal is a gentle scrubbing agent. Metamucil and other psyllium products are too harsh for regular use. Flaxseeds provide the benefit of omega-3 oils and are a nutritious bulking agent that won't damage the inner lining of the small intestines. While psyllium products are fine for a few weeks, chronic use will eventually wear down the tiny finger-like projections in the small intestine, called villi. This is where nutrient absorption occurs, and it is important to not scrub them away. Because of the villi, the surface area of the healthy adult small intestine is about equivalent to the size of a football field. Many older people are malnourished, even if they are obese, because of damage to the villi. So, switch to flaxseeds.

I like to use a coffee-bean-type grinder to break open the seeds and expose the oil—this is the freshest possible flax oil available. Several tablespoons of flax oil several times weekly is also a great way to get omega-3 oils, but I prefer the additional benefits of using the freshly ground seeds.

Talk to Your Health Practitioner

Two common medical problems that can cause mental fogginess are thyroid abnormalities and diabetes. If your foggy thinking is persistent, have your health practitioner check you for these problems, which can then be treated appropriately. It is not uncommon to be overmedicated or experience drug reactions, particularly as we age. The class of drugs used to combat the side effects of other drugs is a multi-*billion* dollar industry. For example, a middle-aged man will be on a beta-blocker for irregular heart rate (when maybe all he needs to do is quit coffee). He then becomes impotent, so is now prescribed Viagra. He's probably also taking Prilosec or some other acid blocker (because he eats so rapidly that his stomach can't break down the food) and maybe a cholesterol-lowering agent, and an aspirin a day. This scenario could apply for women, too—doctors are now giving women Viagra for sexual dysfunction.

What is the effect of all of these drugs in the system? The real answer is that nobody knows exactly what the combined effect of all those different drugs is on your body. Whenever you put something into your mouth that the body does not recognize as digestible food it will, to a certain extent, treat that substance as a foreign material and try to get rid of it. This puts great wear and tear on the immune system and the organs of elimination, especially the kidneys, liver, and skin. I'm not completely against prescription drugs. I just think many people use far too many of them, and I believe this factor contributes to the Alzheimer's epidemic and could also contribute to foggy thinking. If you have been on a prescription drug for four or more years without having your need for that medicine evaluated, check into this right away. Do not assume you need to take a certain drug indefinitely. Even people with insulin-dependent diabetes can lower their need for insulin with a judicious diet.

Miraculous Ginkgo Biloba—The Ancient Plant Medicine

Ginkgo biloba is one of my favorite plant medicines. Ginkgo trees were originally found in Western China, but they now grow around the world in moderate climates and are very resistant to bugs and pollution. A small ginkgo tree was the only plant to survive the Hiroshima atomic bomb, and some trees live to be 1,000 years old. This ancient tree is named biloba, which means two lobes, because its leaves look rather like a heart. Interestingly, given that ginkgo leaves are heart-shaped, it is a wonderful medicine for improving circulation of the blood, especially to the brain. Not only does ginkgo improve blood supply to the brain, it has also been shown to increase the rate of transmission of information through nerve cells. You may read accounts in the press about how ginkgo is not effective for improving cognition, memory, and mental functioning. Don't believe it though, until you have tried it for yourself with a good quality product, standardized to contain 24 percent of the active ingredient (ginkgo flavone glycosides).

Some of the ways ginkgo works to improve blood flow are by mildly thinning the blood and by making red blood cells more flexible. Red blood cells are too large to fit through the smallest vessels in the body, which are numerous in the brain, so these cells need to be able to fold in half to fit through the microcirculation channels (capillary beds). Ginkgo helps red blood cells to fold more easily. Ginkgo also helps to prevent fluid and oxygen loss from damaged and leaky blood vessels by repairing the inner lining of the blood vessels.

Ginkgo is one of the most widely prescribed medicines in Europe, including prescription drugs. It accounts for more than 10 million prescriptions yearly and is used primarily for treating brain and circulation disorders such as headache, short-term memory loss, tinnitus, and vertigo. It is also widely used for the early stages of Alzheimer's disease, and has been shown to successfully delay the deeper cognitive losses that come with the progression of Alzheimer's disease. In some people, myself included, relatively high doses of ginkgo create a photographic memory within several days. (I can personally attest to the value of ginkgo, since it helped me pass my medical board exams.)

In my office, I generally recommend that people with short-term memory problems or foggy thinking start with 240 mg daily of ginkgo, standardized to contain 24 percent ginkgo flavone glycosides. There should be something about 24 percent concentration on the label—don't buy a brand that doesn't claim 24 percent potency. Once the 240 mg daily dose kicks in and you are no longer forgetting your keys or your husband's cell phone number, you can lower the dose to a maintenance level of 40–60 mg daily. You may need to experiment a bit to find the right dose for you.

Very occasionally, the increased blood flow to the brain will cause headaches. I have actually only seen this side effect in one person, and I've prescribed ginkgo to hundreds of people. If you are scheduled for surgery, discontinue ginkgo for a week before and after, because it is a mild blood thinner and could cause excess bleeding. If you are already taking a prescription blood thinner, do not begin ginkgo until you have consulted with a knowledgeable healthcare professional, because you will need to monitor your blood for clotting time and adjust your medicines accordingly.

Don't Forget Exercise (It Helps Everything Else, Too)

It goes almost without saying that regular aerobic exercise will help blood flow to the brain and the rest of the body, and will not only improve foggy thinking, but also digestive function and sleep quality, and most important, it will help you keep a positive attitude.

Treatment Summary

❁ Check your levels of vitamin B_{12} (with a blood test) and the trace mineral zinc (with a blood test, hair analysis, or taste test). If you are low, begin supplementation with 1,000 mcg of vitamin B_{12} daily, preferably a sublingual lozenge form, and take 30 mg of zinc daily in the picolinate form.

❁ Get rid of saturated and hydrogenated fats in your diet. This means Crisco, margarine, cheap salad dressings, and commercially produced baked goods. Replace these bad fats with good fats that actually repair and restore the healthy functioning of the brain and nervous system. Good fats are flax oil, olive oil, and fish oils, especially from coldwater fish, such as salmon and tuna. Take 1–2 tablespoons of flax oil, or even better, 1–3 tablespoons of freshly ground flaxseeds daily in water or juice.

❁ Ginkgo biloba, a plant medicine, standardized to contain 24 percent of the active ingredient, is an extremely effective cure for brain fog. Start with a high dose of 240 mg daily for up to a week until you notice positive effects, then reduce to a maintenance dose, usually 40–60 mg daily. Be sure to use a standardized product.

❁ Daily movement (also known as regular moderate exercise) for an hour daily. You don't have to do the whole hour continuously. Walking briskly, climbing stairs, and housework all count toward the hour of daily movement. This is key in maintaining good blood flow to the brain.

9.

Hair Loss— Some New Ideas

lthough thinning hair is inevitable to some extent as we age, much can be done to keep the shedding to a minimum. Women who have nursed their children, in particular, need to restore key nutrients and maintain high-quality protein intake.

Progesterone May Help, Estrogen May Help

Have you ever noticed how healthy pregnant women just seem to glow—everything about them is glossy and shiny. While they are busy growing a baby, their nails and hair are growing like crazy, too. Typically, the luscious growth of the hair and nails slows way down after the delivery, especially if the devoted mom is nursing, which we hope she is. Nursing is great for the newborn, but it takes a lot of calories to make milk, and generally there is not enough left over for the thick head of hair she enjoyed during pregnancy. Also, progesterone and estrogen levels are much higher during pregnancy. Since both of these female hormones contribute to glossy, healthy hair, it seems quite clear that hormonal changes can affect the health and thickness of our hair.

As with all the other symptoms of hormonal change, I prefer to use hormone replacement as a last resort. This is because I have mild concerns about the absolute safety of natural, bioidentical human hormones while other techniques or nutrients may have beneficial actions with no side effects whatsoever. Nevertheless, a course of progesterone, taken by mouth or by application of a cream to the skin, may be the most effective way to help reverse hair loss in a premenopausal woman who is still menstruating. If your period is regular, and no other method is halting hair shedding, take the progesterone during the second half of your menstrual cycle, about 100 mg daily from day fifteen through thirty. If your cycle is irregular, you could simply vary the progesterone by taking it two weeks on and two weeks off. If you are no longer menstruating and therefore no longer ovulating or producing progesterone, you may find better results with the safest and mildest form of estrogen, estriol (E3). A maximum dose of 5 mg daily may help restore luster to your hair within a few weeks, but watch out for breast tenderness or the return of your menses. Even though bioidentical estriol has never been linked with breast or uterine cancer (in fact, some researchers say E3 protects breast tissue), the theoretical possibility exists. The specter of these cancers certainly should overshadow any longing for a fabulous mane.

Biotin Is the First Best Bet

My favorite over-the-counter remedy for thinning hair is, by far, high-dose biotin. Biotin, a member of the B-vitamin family, is best known for helping heal dry, scaly scalps and easily splitting nails, and for slowing hair loss. The B vitamins are utilized as coenzymes in most parts of the body. They are essential in the proper maintenance of eyes, hair, skin, liver, mouth, and nerves. They are also essential in the production of hormones. A lack of B vitamins can impair fatty-acid synthesis (the good fats).

Although there is no official RDA for biotin, my clinical experience has shown that 100 mcg daily is adequate for people who eat a diet rich in cheese (which I don't generally recommend), organ meats (wild game only is advised) and soybeans. Since not everyone eats like this, I prescribe a higher dose for hair loss. A daily dose of 8,000–10,000 mcg (8–10 mg) will often significantly arrest hair loss within four to six weeks. Continued use may provide ongoing results by stimulating new hair growth. Be aware that antibiotic use can severely decrease biotin levels by destroying biotin-producing gut bacteria. If you have taken more than two rounds of antibiotics in the past several years, you may need to replace biotin levels, especially if antibiotic use was followed by further hair loss. As an aside, researchers from the FDA reported in 1997 that up to 50,000 Americans experience dramatic hair loss after vaccination with the Hepatitis B shot each year.

Plant Medicines

There are several herbal medicines that help with the quality of your hair and may also improve thickness. These include *Equisetum arvense* (horsetail) in tea or capsule form, because of its high mineral content, in particular silica, which is an essential component of strong hair. Supplementing with additional silica may also help, and you can look for shampoos that contain biotin and silica. Avoid conditioners because they tend to contain lots of chemicals that ultimately build up on the hair shaft and make it less healthy. Rosemary may restore hair luster and is also known to help improve memory, in case you're losing your mind as well as your hair! Several Chinese herbs are well known for improving hair thickness, including the ingredients of a traditional combination translated as Seven Treasures for Beautiful Hair. These herbs include angelica (dong quai), ginger, ligusticum, lychee berries, and polygonum. Ginger can be used internally, or rubbed directly onto the scalp. Before washing your hair, cut a piece of fresh ginger root at an angle and rub the juicy part of the cut root into your scalp. Ginger is warming and will increase the blood flow to the scalp. Another excellent way to improve circulation to the scalp is to stand on your head (if you are an expert at yoga) or do a handstand several times weekly.

Headstands

If you've never tried a yoga class—try it. Yoga is a wonderful way to strengthen and stretch all your muscles and improve your circulation. If you are serious about improving the quality of your hair, I recommend building up to the level of holding a headstand for twenty-five to forty slow breaths three to seven times weekly. Note: There can be damage to the neck vertebrae if you do not build up slowly to the headstand. Do not do headstands if you have glaucoma.

Shave and Grow

And here's one more idea that's even more radical than yoga—try shaving your head. In Asian countries, this is widely practiced on the milk hair of infants to encourage it to grow in thick and strong. Most of us have noticed that shaving our leg hair seems to make it grow back thicker.

Self-Massage the Scalp, Work the Acupoints

If you're not ready to shave your head and live under a scarf or incognito in the tropics for a few months, then a nightly head massage will do wonders, not only for your hair but also for your peace of mind. Self-massage is readily available, inexpensive, and you always know just where you need it. The trick is to keep your arms and hands relaxed while massaging. I like to sit comfortably or lie on my back, and place my fingers in my hair then gently pull against it. Move the fingers slightly and squeeze the hands again until the whole scalp has been stimulated. In Chinese medicine, brittle or thin hair is considered a deficiency in the bladder and kidney meridians. The bladder meridian has numerous acupoints on the scalp; treatment with fingertips or acupuncture needles may help stimulate the vital energy needed to create new hair growth.

Treatment Summary

❊ The most important supplement to prevent hair loss and restore hair growth is high-dose biotin. Take 8–10 mg (8,000–10,000 mcg) of this B vitamin in the morning for at least six weeks. No side effects are noted, even at this high dose.

❊ A Chinese patent medicine called Seven Treasures for Beautiful Hair is a combination of several herbal remedies. It is available through my favorite Chinese patent medicine company, Plum Flower, distributed by MayWay Company. I have recently started to use this in my practice, and am getting enthusiastic responses.

❊ Get upside down. Yoga poses offer several elegant options for having your head below your heart. This will greatly increase blood flow, thus oxygen and nutrients, to the scalp and hair follicles. Aim for the expert level of holding a headstand for twenty-five to forty slow breaths, three to seven times weekly. Avoid headstands during your period and if you have glaucoma or a fragile neck.

❊ Finally, avoid toxic chemical exposures, such as inhaling diesel fumes or working overtime in a photo lab. Also, be sure you don't have thyroid or blood-sugar problems, both of which can cause hair loss.

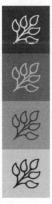

10.

Skin Changes—
How to Prevent Them

Your skin is a fantastic organ that protects your body against injury, bacterial invasion, and the effects of UV light. It is waterproof, and can record touch, changes in temperature, and pain. The skin is largely composed of collagen, which decreases with age. During the first five years after menopause, up to 40 percent of skin collagen is lost. Changes in the skin occur as a result of collagen loss as we age, including brown spots, dryness, easy bruising, and wrinkles. Many of these changes are inevitable, and skin quality is partly genetic, but we can help preserve our skin through a number of natural techniques.

Skin Brushing—Divine

One of my favorite therapies for keeping skin beautiful is skin brushing. This European spa secret involves a daily scrub with a dry, natural bristle, long-handled brush. Don't use a nylon brush. Brush your whole body (except the face) in gentle but firm strokes toward the heart. Don't forget the palms of the hand and soles of the feet. Try this, followed by a cold shower, to replace your morning coffee. I've helped many people give up coffee (and cigarettes) with dry-skin brushing and a cold morning shower. Besides brushing off the layer of dead skin cells that accumulates daily and allowing the skin to breathe easier, skin brushing produces the softest skin imaginable. It is one of the finest of all baths. You make new skin every twenty-four hours, and no soap can wash the skin as clean as the new skin you have under the old. It will be as clean as the blood.

Skin brushing not only removes the top layer of old skin cells, it also stimulates blood circulation and the draining action of our lymphatic system.

The lymphatic system is a whole-body collection of channels, alongside the veins and arteries, which drains the blood of toxins. In terms of surface area, the skin is the largest organ of elimination after the lungs. Your skin is like a third kidney, ridding the body of toxic waste. Healthy skin cells can eliminate two pounds of waste, such as uric and lactic acid, from our bodies daily.

Dry-skin brushing is best accomplished first thing in the morning. Start by scrubbing the palms of the hands, and brush firmly up the arms toward the heart. Then do the soles of the feet and up the legs. Scrub the buttocks, the flanks, up under the breasts, and in a clockwise motion over the abdomen. Use the long handle to get every inch of the back and shoulders. Go over the fatty areas (breasts, butt, hips) one more time until they are pink.

Smaller, fine brushes can be used on your face. First, apply the dry skin brush, and if additional cleaning is required for the face, water is the next choice, then high-fat soaps if the facial skin is truly greasy or grimy. In general, only high-fat soaps (such as black soaps and Neutrogena) are useful in removing grease from the pores. Very coarse facial scrubs such as those with apricot pits are usually too harsh for the delicate skin of the face.

Water—The Universal Solvent

Pure water is the best way to clean your skin. Occasionally you may also need soaps, lotions, or potions, but stick to water when you can. Another way to use water for skin health is by alternating applications of hot and cold water. You can take hip baths, foot baths, or colonics; you can douche, use a hot tub, then a cold plunge, wrap your body in wet towels, or use a whirlpool. Water therapies have been used for centuries by many different cultures, including the Chinese, Egyptians, Greeks, Hebrews, and Hindus, to treat diseases and injuries, and enhance health overall.

An important aspect of water therapy is to alternate between hot and cold applications. The hot water is relaxing and stimulates local blood flow, making your skin turn pink. The cold water is invigorating, and helps pump waste products into the lymph channels and nodes, the body's drainage system. Go back and forth several times between hot and cold, and *always* end on cold, as the final chaser. A very quick, easy way to apply contrast hydrotherapy is to chase your daily bath or shower with at least sixty seconds (that's longer than you might think) of pure cold water. Apply the cold water to the armpits, groin area, along the spine, the bottoms of the feet, and the face. Additionally, if you've washed your hair, a cold rinse on the head is a terrific idea because it flattens the hair follicle, making the light bounce off the hair and giving it a much shinier look. I can often persuade the faint-of-heart to try full-body cold rinses by appealing to their vanity—beautiful hair is a nice fringe benefit. The cold water needs to be at least 60 degrees colder than the hot water. So, if your shower is 100 degrees, the cold chaser needs to be 40 degrees.

Stool Patrol

To have clean shiny skin, your insides also need to be clean. Do what it takes to have a least one well-formed, dark brown, easy-to-pass bowel movement every day. If you tend to have difficulty producing a daily stool, the first order of business is to drink more water. The large intestine is where our precious water is recycled back into the bloodstream. If you aren't drinking enough water your large intestine (which leads directly to the rectum, where the stool is evacuated) may become dry. You can also use gentle natural laxatives, such as aloe vera juice, fennel oil, or senna leaf. It is important to avoid laxative dependence, so work with a nutritionally oriented healthcare provider to find a schedule that will produce perfect bowel movements. My personal favorite bowel stimulant is three tablespoons of freshly ground flaxseeds in diluted pineapple juice or water. Not only does the flax meal gently scrub the large intestine clean (much gentler than psyllium or Metamucil), but it provides fresh omega-3 fatty acids— the best-quality fat your brain and skin could hope for.

If you tend to have loose stools, first make sure you aren't eating contaminated food. More than 5,000 people in the United States die annually of food poisoning, and many more become ill. Often these are children. Avoid fast food; there's nothing good about it. Be sure you are not taking too much magnesium. Some people have a lower tolerance for vitamin C, and can only take a certain amount before their stools become loose. You can also use half a tablespoon of carob powder (in water or rice milk) once or twice daily to firm up the stool. If you have persistent, irregular stool function, consult a healthcare provider soon.

Vitamin E

Vitamin E is an important skin nutrient, and has many other health benefits, as well, to be discussed at greater length in Chapter 14. Vitamin E is naturally present in the skin. Skin that is rich in vitamin E can provide protection against damage caused by the sun's UV rays through a combination of antioxidant and ultraviolet absorptive properties. While a diet rich in vitamin E can increase the total level in the body significantly, only a small portion of this total amount of vitamin E is stored in the skin. Applying vitamin E cream and oils directly to the skin is a very effective way of greatly increasing vitamin E skin levels.

Estrogen

As a last resort, estrogen can be used to maintain healthy skin through the transition to menopause. Estrogen causes the skin to develop a soft smooth texture, but it also creates more blood flow to the skin. This is why women who have higher natural levels of estrogen or who take supplemental estrogen tend to bleed more easily when cut. However, estrogen also increases the chance of forming blood clots in deeper blood vessels. This is the most important reason to stay away from supplemental estrogen. Do not take estrogen in any form if you have a family history of blood-clot formation or strokes. If you do choose estrogen support for your skin, remember to take it along with progesterone if you have a uterus. Also, choose bioidentical estrogens (see Chapter 11 on this topic).

Good Fats

Hormones are fat-based molecules. The precursor of all sex hormones is cholesterol—estrogen, progesterone, testosterone, and thyroxine are structurally similar to cholesterol and use cholesterol as a primary building block. Every single cell in our whole body (there are about 6 billion of them) is made of genetic information surrounded by cell walls. The cell walls are made of two layers of cholesterol, with a layer of water and minerals separating them. This double-cholesterol layer construction protects our cells from drying up and very selectively allows chemicals, hormones, and nutrients in and out of the cell.

As we age and hormonal function changes, the amount of cholesterol we produce is also reduced. The strength and flexibility of our cells are at risk unless we choose to eat healthy fats and restrict our consumption of bad fats. It becomes even more critical as we age to choose healthy fats in our diet to maintain healthy skin and healthy insides, too. Both dry and oily skin conditions are indicative of not enough good fats (from borage, olive, and evening primrose oils, coldwater fish, and flaxseeds) and too many bad fats (any fat that is solid at room temperature). All fats and oils, including nuts, must be kept refrigerated to prevent further rancidity. High quality oils, such as flax oil, should never be used for cooking, but only in salad dressings or as a butter substitute over hot oatmeal or vegetables.

Cholesterol

Do not attempt no-fat diets even though your cholesterol may be creeping up a few points. A no-fat diet will ruin your skin. Why do cholesterol levels often go up at menopause, and just before it? For two reasons: First, our livers may not be as efficient at breaking down and excreting excess cholesterol as they once were, especially the bad LDL cholesterol (LDL goes into the bloodstream and gets deposited there, while the good HDL comes back to the liver from the blood and is broken down or used as fuel). Second, we make less cholesterol as we age, and the body hangs onto it more tightly. Chapter 21 provides more information about cholesterol and cholesterol testing.

Liver Spots

This leads to my final suggestion for beautiful skin—keep your liver working well. Those flat brown spots that increasingly appear on the skin as we age are referred to as liver spots, and I believe there is some truth to that concept. The liver is a major detoxification organ, and the overflow of wastes it cannot handle may be eliminated through the skin. One good example of this is jaundice from hepatitis. With an acute liver infection such as hepatitis the liver can no longer efficiently recycle bile, its most important secretion. The bile backs up in the blood and colors the skin and whites of the eyes a yellowish color. (The French word for yellow is jaune.) One of my favorite approaches to helping the bile flow smoothly through the liver is to eat beets—fresh, organic, cubed, steamed, and lightly marinated beets, with good quality olive oil and a little balsamic vinegar. They'll stay good in a Mason jar in the fridge for nearly two weeks. Eat four to six pieces (half a cup) daily to improve liver function. The deep healing pigments in the beets will stain your stool and urine, so don't be alarmed if you notice this.

Another way to protect your liver is to avoid solvents, which include alcoholic beverages, hours with your arms in photography chemicals, paint thinner, and standing right next to the gas pump. You may not need to completely abandon drinking alcohol if you drink moderately and tests show that your liver function is good. However, if you don't drink, you're likely to live a longer, healthier life. Chapter 15 has a more complete discussion on liver cleansing.

Treatment Summary

❋ Skin *brushing is the finest way to cleanse your skin. Use a natural bristle brush on dry skin first thing every morning.*

❋ Do *contrast hydrotherapy daily, alternating between hot- and cold-water applications to your skin. Always end with a cold chaser. The easiest way to do this is in the shower—rinse with pure cold water, especially under the armpits, the groin area, the mid-back, and the head (if you are washing your hair).*

❋ Maintain *optimal bowel function, which means a dark brown, well-formed, easy-to-pass bowel movement at least once every day. If you tend to be constipated, your first consideration is drinking more pure water. Start your drinking water in the morning so you form a taste for this wonderful cleansing beverage early in the day.*

❋ *Vitamin E is a critical nutrient for the skin, more important than vitamin C at this time of life. Get a reputable brand of vitamin E (my favorite is Carlson Laboratories) and take 400 IU daily. You may need 800 IU if you live in a dry climate or if your skin is particularly dry, fair, or thin. You can also apply vitamin E cream and oils directly to your skin.*

PART TWO

Marvelous and Incredibly Useful Natural Substances

11.

Bioidentical Hormones

As a physician, I have consistently believed that hormone replacement therapy should be the last resort when treating women as they transition through menopause. The results of recent scientific research have supported my position. The safety and even the benefits of hormonal drugs have been called into question. In July 2002, the Women's Health Initiative prematurely halted its huge study of more than 16,000 women taking the hormone Prempro (a standard dose of a form of estrogen plus a synthetic form of progesterone) because of significant increases in blood clots, breast cancer, heart disease, and strokes. The results were drawn from the federally funded series of clinical trials begun in 1997 to look at the effect of conventional estrogen and progesterone on menopausal women. The Prempro arm of the trial was halted three years short of the eight-year study design because of higher incidences of disease in women taking the hormones, and because of an accompanying *lack of any benefits* from hormone therapy. These findings, which received wide press attention, were officially announced on July 9, 2002 by the National Institutes of Health, the major sponsor of the WHI trials, and were published in the May 8, 2003 issue of *The New England Journal of Medicine*.

At the time of the study, Prempro was the best-selling drug on the market. The 6 million women using it have now been advised to stop, because it appears that the progestin, a synthetic progesterone-like compound, is the culprit in the increase of potentially fatal side effects.

The women taking these hormones were led to believe that the quality and length of their lives would be improved. It was a shock for them and their doctors to find out the opposite might be true, or that they might not make any difference at all. The results apply only to long-term use, not to women taking HRT short-term for relief of hot flashes. Nor do they apply to women taking only estrogen. If you have been taking the hormone combo (Prempro, which is Premarin plus Provera), you can stop right away, but you might be more comfortable if you wean yourself from it. If you have been on this hormone combination for five years or more, it is very important that you stop as soon as possible.

These results do not mean that hormones are always risky and should never be taken. Bioidentical hormones have been shown to carry most of the benefits and no evidence of the risks of the patentable hormones. Let me explain.

The "Real" Thing—Not "New and Improved"

All prescribed hormones, natural or otherwise, are synthesized in a laboratory. We couldn't ethically extract human hormones from humans for resale, but scientists began to figure out how to create all sorts of naturally occurring chemicals, including hormones, in the laboratory as early as the turn of the century. The fact that these hormones are synthetic is not the problem. The problem is that *most* prescribed hormones are not exactly identical to the natural estrogen, progesterone, and testosterone molecules in women's bodies. Why not? Drug companies cannot patent a naturally occurring substance, so they need to modify it a little biochemically in order to patent it and make it into a best-selling drug. They sell these chemicals, which look similar to human hormones but are not identical to them, at highly inflated prices because the research and development required to bring them to market is enormously expensive. Some estimates state that bringing a new drug to market costs, on the average, $450 million. Of course, the drug companies want to recover their costs and get a good return on their investment.

If hormone therapy does prove to be necessary for your health and comfort, your other choice is to find a doctor who works with bioidentical hormones. The bioidentical hormones (sometimes abbreviated as nHRT for natural HRT) are also created in a laboratory, but they are chemically *identical* to human hormones. These bioidentical hormones are not patentable because they are exactly the same as the estrogen, progesterone, and testosterone hormones that are made in your body. The irony here is that although these bioidentical substances, made mostly from plant sources, cost less to produce than their pharmaceutically altered cousins, the drug companies would rather spend millions on *non*-identical products so they can patent them, control the market, and charge whatever they want. The Europeans, who are offered a national healthcare plan, use bioidentical hormones widely because they are safer, less expensive, and work better. They can be purchased in this country through specialty pharmacies.

Another aspect of the bioidentical versus patent hormone controversy is the source material for the synthetic hormones. Bioidentical hormones are generally made from plant sources, most commonly soy or Mexican wild yam. The patent hormones (such as Prempro) are often made from the urine of pregnant animals, often mares (hence the name Premarin). Some conventionally trained doctors actually believe that Premarin is natural because it comes from a horse. It may be natural for a horse, but certainly not for a woman.

Although I believe the bad side effects of Prempro and similar drugs derive largely from the fact that these hormones are not bioidentical, no hormone therapy can be considered completely safe until this is proven. That is why I always turn to hormone therapy as a last resort when helping women through their perimenopausal and menopausal symptoms.

Before detailing the risks of hormones, I'd like to give you a little history on the subject. Estrogen replacement therapy (ERT) was aggressively promoted to doctors, doctors' wives, and other women during the 1960s. The manufacturers of Premarin, which is a non-bioidentical, synthetic estrogen derived from pregnant mares' urine, commissioned a book by Dr. Robert A. Wilson, *Feminine Forever.* As I'm sure you can guess, that insidious little book is all about taking estrogen so you'll always be sexually appealing to your husband, have lovely skin, keep your breasts perky, age more slowly, and "avoid the psychological problems that accompany the change of life." I know women who remember Tupperware-style parties, complete with records and glossy photos, given by doctors' wives to promote estrogen within their social circles. No surprise, the tactic worked. By 1975, Premarin was one of the top five most prescribed drugs in the United States.

Unfortunately, Premarin causes endometrial cancer. The endometrium is the lining of the womb. It normally sheds monthly as a menstrual period, and should not be artificially stimulated. Some scientists figured out that the risk of endometrial cancer would go away if a progesterone-like substance was added to the Premarin. ERT (estrogen replacement therapy) became HRT (hormone replacement therapy, incorporating both estrogen and progestin), the standard prescription for women with a womb. The market started to revive.

Hormone Supplementation as a Preventative

The pharmaceutical scientists then began to promote other uses for the combination drug. "Take it to prevent osteoporosis, take it to prevent heart disease, take it to prevent Alzheimer's," they said. The drug reps tried to avoid mentioning that adding the progestin (fake progesterone) didn't make the breast-cancer risk go away but instead made it worse. The increased risk of breast cancer from taking hormones was pretty much ignored as were the other risks for HRT use, including abnormal bleeding resulting in hysterectomy, asthma, liver and gallbladder disease, lupus, and ovarian cancer. Women who use hormones are eight times more likely to have abnormal bleeding than women who go through menopause without hormone therapy. Remember, menopause is a *natural* transition in a woman's life—not a disease.

More recently, we have learned that HRT does nothing to prevent heart disease and may even increase the occurrence of certain types of cardiovascular problems such as blood clots and strokes. The claims that HRT prevents dementia have not been substantiated, and the initial research claiming that women who take HRT are less likely to become senile turns out to have more to do with the socioeconomic status of the women taking HRT. Women who have regular checkups and are most concerned about their looks as they age are likely to be wealthier women with more leisure time. These women are more likely to read for study and pleasure, travel, volunteer their time for charitable causes, and in general, use their brains. Although there is certainly a genetic component to Alzheimer's disease, using your brain vigorously prolongs the liveliness and fortitude of your mental capacity. I mention this largely because women from every socioeconomic class need to know that reading and studying topics of interest will delay brain aging. Almost every community has a library. The brain is like a muscle, so, as they say, use it or lose it.

HRT Does Not Prevent:

✼ Alzheimer's disease

✼ Heart disease

✼ Memory loss

✼ Psychological problems

✼ Reduced sexual desire or responsiveness

✼ Urinary incontinence

✼ Wrinkles or other natural signs of aging

Reasons to Avoid or Discontinue Hormone Therapy

There is increased risk for:

- ❦ Benign breast problems, such as cysts
- ❦ Blood clots
- ❦ Breast, ovarian, or uterine cancer
- ❦ Gallbladder disease
- ❦ Heart attacks
- ❦ High blood pressure
- ❦ Kidney disease associated with fluid retention

- ❦ Migraines
- ❦ Pregnancy (could harm the fetus)
- ❦ Seizure disorder
- ❦ Severe liver disease, such as hepatitis C
- ❦ Strokes
- ❦ Unexplained vaginal bleeding
- ❦ Uterine fibroids

The Quick Guide to Bioidentical (But Not Customized) Hormone Replacement Therapy (HRT)

- **Alora.** Estrogen only. Transdermal patch, completely synthetic but bioidentical

- **Climara.** Estrogen only. Transdermal patch, synthesized from soy

- **Estrace.** Estrogen only. Oral administration or vaginal cream, synthesized from soy and yams

- **Estraderm.** Estrogen only. Transdermal patch, synthesized from Mexican yams

- **Estring.** Estrogen only. Vaginal ring, synthesized from Mexican yams

- **Fempatch.** Estrogen only. Transdermal patch, completely synthetic but bioidentical

- **Vivelle.** Estrogen only. Transdermal patch, synthesized from Mexican yams

- **Crinone.** Progesterone only. Vaginal gel, synthesized from Mexican yams

- **Prometrium.** Progesterone only. Oral, synthesized from Mexican yams

- **Androderm.** Testosterone only. Transdermal patch, synthesized from soy

- **Androgel.** Testosterone only. Transdermal patch, synthesized from yams or soy

- **Testoderm.** Testosterone only. Transdermal patch, completely synthetic but bioidentical

Bioidentical Hormones in Hormone Therapy

As you can see from "The Quick Guide to Bioidentical Hormone Replacement Therapy (HRT)" on page 85, prescription bioidentical single hormones are available.

How do the drug companies make money on them? Although they can't patent the main ingredient, which is the bioidentical hormone, they are able to patent the fillers, binders, and dyes used in the making of the pills and creams. For example, Prometrium, a bioidentical progesterone, is a little round ball covered in a red sugar coating. Because the shape and color of the pill are proprietary to the manufacturer the entire pill can be marketed as a unique product. You can use these prescription items if you must, but I strongly urge you to consider using a compounding pharmacist to find the exact right blend of estrogens, progesterone (if needed), and testosterone (if needed) for you instead. Compounding pharmacists are a wonderful resource and can make up a custom formula using bioidentical hormones (see the Resources section).

There is one more issue I would like to discuss at this point: the definition of estrogen. Everyone has heard of estrogen, but are we all thinking the same thing when we read this word? Any discussion in the popular press about estrogen is usually referring to estradiol, or E2, but a good understanding of all the estrogen hormones will help you make the right choice for your health and comfort.

There are three major forms of estrogen in the female body: E1, or estrone (the "one" in estrone represents 1); E2, estradiol (dio meaning 2); and E3, estriol (tri meaning 3). Of the three estrogens, E1 is the strongest and potentially the most cancer-causing, which is why it is not often used. Estradiol, E2, is the most commonly used form of estrogen. It is almost as strong (with positive effects on bone, negative effects on the uterus) as E1, perhaps because some of it converts to E1 in the small intestine. Estriol, E3, is the weakest estrogen, but it seems to have positive effects on bone and skin without increasing the risks for blood clots, breast, or uterine cancers. Some holistically oriented doctors like to use E3 alone for perimenopausal and menopausal problems, and some prefer to use a combination of E2 and E3 (Bi-Est). When first researched, Estriol (E3) was considered too weak to have any biological effect. Fortunately researchers in China, Europe, and Japan continued to study E3, and from their research it looks as though E3 alone does help increase bone mineral density, and reduce hot flashes, vaginal dryness, and total cholesterol and triglyceride levels.

Because the human body makes these three types of estrogen, another line of thinking promotes the idea of using all three, in a ratio similar to that found in the body. Doctors who use a triple-estrogen-compounded formula (Tri-Est) tend to use the three estrogens in a 10:10:80 ratio, since this is what has been discovered in human urine. More recently, however, blood studies suggest that a more realistic ratio would be less than 10 percent each of E1 and E2, and 90 percent or more of E3. I mostly use Bi-Est (E2 and E3) when indicated for my menopausal patients.

If you do choose to use hormones, I hope you will choose bioidentical hormones, blended specifically for your needs and risks. If you do not have a uterus, you may not need to use progesterone at all. Its use as a hormone is principally for sustaining a pregnancy, but we know that progesterone receptors exist throughout the body, and not just in the uterus, so another purpose for this hormone may be discovered in the future. We do know that progesterone is only secreted in the female body after ovulation. If you have a uterus, you will need to use progesterone if using estrogen to prevent uterine cancer. Pharmaceutical, nonbioidentical progesterone (progestin) will increase the risk of breast cancer that comes with taking patented hormones, but I believe that bioidentical hormones pose virtually no risk, especially the weak estrogen, E3, although this idea has yet to be definitively proven.

Finally, if you are still menstruating regularly and choose to use hormone replacement therapy you will, of course, need to use progesterone along with estrogen, but only use the progesterone in the second half of your menstrual cycle. If you are no longer bleeding regularly you are advised to use the same dose of estrogen and progesterone daily throughout the month, to avoid stimulating regular menses again. If you *want* to reestablish a regular period, that may be possible with a hormone therapy that mimics the menstrual cycle: estrogen high in midcycle, followed by a surge of progesterone. Work with your doctor to help figure out these details. This book is primarily intended to help you manage menopause naturally, *without* hormones.

EFFECTS OF ESTROGEN AND PROGESTERONE EXCESS OR DEFICIENCY

ESTROGEN EXCESS	PROGESTERONE EXCESS*	ESTROGEN DEFICIENCY	PROGESTERONE DEFICIENCY
Anxiety	Breast swelling	Bone loss	Anxiety
Bleeding changes	Breast tenderness	Foggy thinking	Depressed mood
Breast tenderness	Depressed mood	Hot flashes	Foggy thinking
Cyclical headaches	Sleepiness	Incontinence	Hot flashes
Hot flashes	Slowed digestion	Memory lapses	Low libido
Irritability		Night sweats	Memory lapses
Mood swings		Sleep disturbances	Night sweats
Nervousness		Vaginal dryness	Sleep disturbances
Night sweats			Vaginal dryness
Sleep disturbances			
Water retention			
Weight gain			

Rare, except with oversupplementation

Table courtesy of Transitions for Health Women's Institute, Portland, OR.

12.

Antioxidants, Bioflavonoids, and Vitamin C

This chapter could also be titled "Whole Foods—The Ultimate Natural Supplements." Ideally, all of our nutritional needs would be met by consuming a diet of whole foods. A whole food is a food made of only one ingredient that grew in the soil fairly recently. (Can you visualize a field of Twinkies?) The most vibrant, radiant, and life-giving of the whole foods are, without question, fruits and vegetables. Fruits and vegetables are loaded with antioxidants, bioflavonoids, and vitamin C. And that's not all. They have calories, enzymes, fiber, minerals, and moisture. I recommend that all adults consume at least two servings (one cup) of green vegetables (the darker the better), at least one serving (one-half cup) of orange vegetables, and at least one serving (one-half cup) of whole fruit every day. I'm not the only one who recommends regular consumption of fruits and vegetables. The American Cancer Society, the American Heart Association, and the National Institutes of Health all recommend five to nine servings of fruits and vegetables daily. Try to eat fruits and vegetables when they are in season.

If you don't like vegetables, you may need to be creative about getting them into your diet regularly. For example, you can dip raw vegetables (carrots, celery, sliced peppers) into bean paste, guacamole, or a homemade cream sauce. You can also make hearty soups with lots of vegetables. One of my favorite soups is Molly Katzen's "Gypsy Soup" in *The Moosewood Cookbook*, which calls for a base of chopped onion and tomatoes, plus two green vegetables, such as celery, chopped kale, green pepper, or peas, and two orange vegetables, such as carrots, squash, sweet potatoes, or yams, all spiced with basil, cinnamon, oregano, turmeric, salt, and pepper.

Antioxidants

Antioxidants are among the marvelous natural substances found in fruits and vegetables. It's important to understand that while oxygen is essential for life, too much oxygen exposure is not a good thing. When metals containing iron are exposed to excess oxygen, they rust. Rust is an example of oxidative damage, and the aging process is basically due to oxidative damage. One of the most destructive forms of oxidative damage is the "rusting" of fatty tissues, technically called lipid peroxidation, which can happen in our arteries, our organs, and our skin. Because fat is a part of many tissues of the body (the brain, the inner lining of arteries, the organs, and the skin), these parts of the body are subject to lipid peroxidation.

Most oxidative damage occurs within the body, but exposure to acrylic paints, alcohol, anesthetics, barbecued foods, cigarette smoke and other air pollutants, cleaning fluids, coffee, fried foods, furniture polish, pesticides, and petroleum-based products all hasten the permanent destruction of our tissues. Avoid these substances. Another important way to protect against excessive "fat rust" is to consume whole foods containing the antioxidant vitamins A, C, and E and the minerals selenium and zinc. However, the antioxidants we get from our foods are often not enough to counteract the ever-increasing burden that pollution puts on our immune system. It is wise for anyone over the age of thirty-five to supplement with up to 20,000 IU of vitamin A (beta-carotene is the optimal form), 5 grams (5,000 mg) of vitamin C, 800 IU of vitamin E, 200 mcg of selenium, and 30 mg of zinc daily. If you regularly eat fruits and vegetables, you don't need to take vitamin and mineral supplements every day. Some of the most powerful food antioxidants include the berries (especially bilberry and blueberry), dark leafy greens, dark chocolate, grapes, and soy products. "Chocolate?" you ask, eyes lighting up. Just to clarify, *dark*—not milk—chocolate confers that benefit, but the downside is, of course, the fat and the sugar. Unsweetened, organic, dark cocoa powder is really the health food, but to eat chocolate without guilt, choose a dark, organic Fair Trade variety. Most health food stores carry organic chocolate (Endangered Species Chocolate Company, Green & Black's Organic Fair Trade Chocolate, Newman's, Rapunzel), and it's well worth it to avoid the heavy pesticide residue.

Bioflavonoids

Bioflavonoids are another group of plant substances that protect against oxidative damage. This remarkable group of pigments provides the beautiful coloration of flowers, fruits, and vegetables. Colorful and visually pleasing foods are usually healthy choices, but don't be fooled by artificial food dyes. (If it's bright orange and looks like an orange, go for it. If it's bright orange and looks like a blob of Jell-O, just say no.) Besides providing color, bioflavonoids are antiallergenic, anticarcinogenic, anti-inflammatory, and antiviral. Much of the therapeutic activity of plant medicines is due to the action of bioflavonoids. More than 400 bioflavonoids have been classified, with such names as anthocyanidin, catechin, hesperidin, ipriflavone, isoflavone, rutin, and so on.

One of the ways bioflavonoids work is to strengthen the human vascular system. This means they protect our heart and arteries and reduce the potential for clotting. In fact, Dr. John Folts, who helped popularize the use of aspirin for preventing heart attacks, has written that flavonoids may work even better than aspirin. Milk thistle, a plant with a long history of use in treating liver diseases, contains bioflavonoids specific for liver repair. Ginkgo biloba, used to improve blood flow to the brain, contains flavonoids specific to the central nervous system (the brain and spinal cord). Another way bioflavonoids protect our health is by increasing the positive effects of vitamin C.

Vitamin C

Thanks to the decades of study by the late Dr. Linus Pauling, two-time Nobel-Prize winner for his work on vitamin C, we now have a deep appreciation of the importance of ascorbic acid, the chemical name for vitamin C, in human health. If I had to choose *one* supplement only for the rest of my life, it would be vitamin C without a doubt. That's because vitamin C is the main nutrient required for tissue repair. Vitamin C heals wounds, encourages healthy bone and tooth maintenance, and helps regulate important minerals in the body, especially iron and calcium. Without vitamin C our bodies cannot repair worn-out cartilage (present in all our joints). The production of collagen, which holds our skin and flesh together, is dependent on vitamin C.

Because vitamin C deteriorates rapidly when exposed to prolonged heat, the best way to get adequate vitamin C in the diet is to eat fruits and lightly steamed vegetables that are rich in this nutrient every day. Good choices include cabbage, citrus fruits, colored peppers, leafy green vegetables, strawberries, sweet potatoes, and tomatoes. We suffer continual microdamage to our tissues because of breathing, eating, moving, thinking, and all of our other physical and mental functions, but our bodies heal at night as we sleep. Vitamin C is the principal ingredient in the nightly repair of human tissue, which is largely carried out by dynamic protein units called enzymes. Unlike most other higher mammals, however, humans do not manufacture their own vitamin C. Many older people who do not get proper nutrition are deficient in vitamin C, which hastens their aging.

The importance of vitamin C became known when the globe was being explored by large sailing vessels. Scurvy, the famous disease caused by inadequate vitamin C intake, became rampant during long voyages. Scurvy is not pretty—the teeth rot, the skin gets saggy, flaky, and gray, and the whole digestive system, from the gums to the rectum, bleeds. Eventually it was determined that fresh fruits and vegetables, particularly citrus, could prevent this disease. British sailors were called limeys because the men were ordered to suck on limes while at sea.

Stress depletes the body of vitamin C, and so does a cold or flu. Much of the vitamin C in our bodies is stored inside white blood cells, the workhorses of the immune system. When a bug or an allergic compound comes along (the antigen), certain white blood cells (B cells) tag the antigen with a mirror image of itself (called an antibody), and other white blood cells (macrophages) dump vitamin C and enzymes on the antigen-antibody complex, killing it, digesting it, and preparing it for removal from the body.

Too much vitamin C can cause diarrhea, so work up to your optimal dose slowly. I recommend starting with 500 mg daily, then increasing by 500 mg each day until you experience loose stools. Then cut back by about 20 percent. During periods of illness increase your vitamin C and fluids, and reduce your intake of solid food. Avoid high doses of vitamin C just before a scheduled surgery, because it is a mild blood thinner.

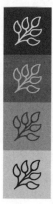

13.

The B Vitamins

Long known as the antistress vitamins, a good B-multi can do wonders to restore calm and sanity to a harried lifestyle. Without B vitamins, your nervous system cannot function properly, and this includes thinking straight. B vitamins also play an important role in helping to prevent heart disease (discussed at greater length in Chapter 21). Furthermore, specific B vitamins are essential for converting amino acids, carbohydrates, and fats into protein, the building block for tissue repair. There are several B vitamins, and while it is best to supplement with a product that contains all the Bs, sometimes also taking supplemental higher doses of a specific B vitamin may be a good idea. If you eat meat and digest it well, you are probably not deficient in B vitamins, although increased doses may help with specific problems, for example, extra B_6 for PMS. Vegans (strict vegetarians) will have a more difficult time ingesting sufficient B vitamins although grains, legumes, prunes, and raisins do contain small amounts. High heat, as used in processed foods, destroys B vitamins. The following paragraphs will briefly introduce each of the B vitamins.

Vitamin B_1 (Thiamine)

Vitamin B_1 is a critical nutrient that allows the brain to function correctly, and it is required for memory. In the 1940s, large oral doses and injectable vitamin B_1 were used for pain control, for example, to treat migraines, or to reduce pain from amputated limbs or dental extractions. This was discontinued as more effective analgesics were developed. Vitamin B_1 is depleted by alcohol and is the most common B-vitamin deficiency in alcoholics. A deficiency of

B_1 causes Wernicke-Korsakoff syndrome, a pronounced and irreversible dementia, and beri-beri, a nasty complex of heart swelling and problems with nerve endings, especially in the legs. Around 50 mg daily is generally sufficient for supplementation.

Vitamin B_2 (Riboflavin)

Vitamin B_2 is important in energy production because it helps convert carbohydrates to protein. It also allows for the recycling of an important antioxidant, glutathione. B_2 is responsible for making the urine turn bright yellow. Some people with migraines have been cured by taking 400 mg daily of B_2. A deficiency of this vitamin causes the corners of the mouth to crack and become infected, and may also contribute to a scaly, greasy dandruff called seborrhea. Around 50 mg daily is sufficient for supplementation.

Vitamin B_3 (Niacin, or Nicotinic Acid)

Vitamin B_3 is an antioxidant and helps convert both carbohydrates and fats into protein. It helps with many detoxification pathways in the liver, and aids in regulating blood sugar. It can lower bad cholesterol and raise good cholesterol very effectively. It has been used in high doses to control schizophrenia. Doses greater than 100 mg daily will cause flushing of the skin, which is temporary but can be annoying, and it can exaggerate hot flashes. Look for B_3 in the form of inositol hexaniacinate if you don't like the flush but want to take niacin to lower your cholesterol or as part of a multivitamin for overall health. Usually 100 mg of B_3 daily is plenty and won't cause a flush. Avoid sustained-release niacin, since this form has been documented to cause liver problems. Severe B_3 deficiency causes pellagra, a triad of dementia, diarrhea, and peeling skin.

Vitamin B_5 (Pantothenic Acid)

You may not have heard of vitamin B_5, but it is very important for proper adrenal gland function. The adrenal gland, you may remember, is not only responsible for the body's fight or flight reaction, via adrenaline, it also secretes the major natural anti-inflammatory substance, cortisol, which, in excess, causes problems with the metabolism of fat and sugar. Since a properly functioning adrenal gland is critical to the perimenopausal woman, pantothenic acid is perhaps the most important of the B vitamins during this time. Sometimes a B_5 deficiency shows up as anxiety attacks, burning feet, and vague abdominal discomfort. A dose of 50 mg daily is enough to restore proper adrenal function, but you also have to quit coffee and avoid high stress situations.

Vitamin B_6 (Pyridoxine)

Vitamin B_6 is important in helping to prevent anemia, which can occur with heavier menstrual bleeding in the perimenopausal phase leading up to menopause. B_6 works with folic acid (another B vitamin) to prevent neural tube defects in fetuses. A deficiency of B_6 in infants can cause seizures. A massive prolonged overdose can, paradoxically, cause nerve damage, but that is very rare. B_6 is critical to the body's production of red blood cells, anti-inflammatory agents, and for converting amino acids to protein. It is critical for normal hormonal function. Sometimes B_6 supplementation can cure PMS, and it can greatly help carpal tunnel syndrome, as well as rheumatoid arthritis in the hands. Adequate intake of B_6 will also help with healing skin and repairing nerve damage. Along with B_{12} and folic acid, B_6 can also help to prevent heart disease. Birth control pills are notorious for depleting B_6 levels, which may be why the pill causes depression, fatigue, irritability, and lethargy. Supplementation with B_6 may be very effective in controlling skin eruptions in women with cyclic acne. Generally, 50–100 mg daily is enough.

Vitamin B_{12} (Cyano- or Hydroxy-Cobalamin)

Vitamin B_{12} helps prevent pernicious anemia, which, unlike iron-deficient anemia from blood loss, is caused by red blood cells that become too large to pass into the smallest blood vessels. Vitamin B_{12} will help make the abnormal red blood cells more flexible and appropriate in size. Along with B_6, vitamin B_{12} protects against heart disease and carpal tunnel syndrome. It works with folic acid to prevent nerve damage in fetuses. This is especially important to consider if you are an older woman desiring pregnancy. Only tiny doses are needed daily (100–1,000 mcg) but without this level, the hormonal, immune, and nervous systems cannot function properly. If you eat dairy products, eggs, fish, or meat, you probably get plenty of B_{12}. But as we age, *absorption* becomes a problem. If lab tests suggest you are low in B_{12} despite an adequate diet, you may need to supplement with under-the-tongue lozenges (sublingual troches) or intramuscular injections for a while. Vegetarians should supplement with B_{12} and try to regularly eat fermented foods such as kim-chee (like sauerkraut) and miso, which can provide B_{12} from the bacteria that cause the fermentation.

Biotin

Biotin is a B vitamin that helps the body effectively use fat and protein for energy. Biotin is manufactured by healthy bacteria in our intestines, and prolonged antibiotic use, which depletes these, will lead to biotin deficiency. Deficiency signs include a shiny tongue without a coating and skin problems. Biotin has been shown to help improve blood-sugar control in diabetics. It is an important supplement for immune health and is very useful for female hair loss. I have helped many patients improve their hair and nail growth and quality with high-dose biotin, 8–10 grams (8,000–10,000 mcg) daily. Normally, supplementation of 100 mcg daily is adequate.

Folic Acid

Although folic acid is not a B vitamin, it works synergistically with many of the B vitamins. It is naturally present in leafy green vegetables and liver. It helps protect against precancerous changes in the cells of the uterine cervix (cervical dysplasia), and along with vitamins B_6 and B_{12}, protects against heart disease, nerve damage, and neural tube defects in fetuses. A daily dose of 400 mcg is protective.

14.
Vitamin E

Vitamin C and the B vitamins are water-soluble. Water soluble vitamins dissolve readily in fluids and are easily excreted through the normal channels of elimination in the body: sweat, urine, and fecal matter. The fat-soluble vitamins do not dissolve readily in water, are better absorbed when taken with dietary fat, and are usually marketed in gel caps. The four main oil-soluble vitamins are A, D, E, and K. This chapter focuses on the health benefits of vitamin E for the perimenopausal woman, but information about the other fat-soluble vitamins is available elsewhere in the book.

Vitamin E Benefits

Vitamin E is a natural skin protectant. Skin contains vitamin E and vitamin E receptors. Skin rich in vitamin E will have natural protection against damage caused by the sun's ultraviolet (UV) rays. Applying vitamin E cream and oils directly to the skin is a very effective way to increase the levels of vitamin E in the skin.

Vitamin E also plays a critical role in protection from heart disease. Women are catching up with men in heart disease deaths, so it cannot be considered a man's disease any longer. There are many risk factors for premature (before age sixty-five) death from heart disease, such as being overweight, having high blood pressure, being sedentary, having high cholesterol levels, and high homocysteine (a marker of B vitamin status) levels. However, the World Health Organization has found that vitamin E status was more important than these as a risk factor in heart-disease death. In more recent findings, the Cambridge Heart Antioxidant study was stopped early, when vitamin E was shown to be so effective in controlling angina (chest pain caused by a narrowing of the heart vessels) in the vitamin-E group that the researchers felt it was unethical to deprive the placebo group any longer.

Other benefits of vitamin E include reduction of menstrual and arthritic pain. As little as 400 IU of vitamin E just a few days before the expected menses can significantly reduce menstrual pain. However, I advise all my patients over the age of forty to take 400 IU daily, preferably with a meal that contains some fat, to enhance absorption. About 1.5 IU of vitamin E is equivalent to one milligram of alpha-tocopherol, the chemical name for the naturally occurring vitamin.

Vitamin E is a potent antioxidant, so it helps to slow the aging process and enhance repair of body tissues. The fat-soluble vitamins can be thought of as prohormones, because hormones are also fatty compounds. Besides being a wonderful nutrient for the brain, heart, and skin, vitamin E can extend the action of hormones in our system. For example, instead of a progesterone cream or an estrogen suppository for vaginal dryness, vitamin E is extremely effective taken internally (about 400 IU daily, but triple that dose is safe) and can also be applied externally to the vaginal tissues. When vitamin E was discovered in the mid-twentieth century it was dubbed the sex vitamin, because it was thought to increase male virility and help lubricate the female sexual response. We now know that the benefits of vitamin E extend well beyond these claims. Numerous studies have supported vitamin E supplementation to help control heart disease, improve athletic stamina, protect the lungs against air pollution, protect red blood cells, and as mentioned before, slow the process of oxidative cell damage and therefore retard the aging process.

Studies consistently show that those who live past 100 have higher than average vitamin E levels. This might be, in part, because vitamin E is also essential for normal immune function. Vitamin E supplementation has been shown to enhance immune response and resistance to disease. For example, healthy older subjects who received the hepatitis-B vaccine series had a significantly better response if they had been supplementing with at least 200 IU of vitamin E daily in the previous year. A better response was measured by higher levels of antibodies to hepatitis B in their blood after the vaccination series, which means their immune systems were more prepared to fight a possible exposure to the virus.

Forms and Sources of Vitamin E

There is some controversy about the best form of vitamin E. Some companies claim that the synthetic version of vitamin E, which can be made to contain various forms of the vitamin, is superior. Clinical experience leads me to believe that the natural form, d-alpha-tocopherol (the primary of four principal tocopherols), is more readily absorbed than the synthetic varieties (for example, dl-alpha-tocopherol), and therefore more useful to humans. The human placenta in a pregnant woman's uterus has been shown to be four times more likely to absorb natural vitamin E than the synthetic type.

Almonds, sunflower seeds, and sweet potatoes are high in vitamin E, but to get just 100 IU of vitamin E you would need to eat at least one and a third cups of sunflower seeds, two and a quarter cups of almonds, or six and a half cups of sweet potatoes. Therefore, supplementation with a high-quality vitamin E product is generally more efficient.

I have used Carlson Laboratory's vitamin E for nearly twenty years because I consistently see excellent results. For example, in my first (and only) pregnancy at age forty-two, I took 400–800 IU of Carlson vitamin E almost daily and regularly applied Carlson's vitamin E oil from neck to knees during the third trimester, and I did not get a single stretch mark on my body. After an easy delivery in my own home (my daughter was born, as planned, on the kitchen floor), I regularly applied Carlson vitamin E to my nipples, which protected them enough to allow me to nurse her for more than three years.

Vitamin E Supplementation Issues

If you need to supplement with iron because of iron-deficiency anemia, take your iron at least eight hours apart from your vitamin E supplement. Iron is an oxidant and can destroy antioxidants like vitamin E. Food sources of vitamin E are not destroyed by iron, however, just as food sources of iron, such as romaine lettuce, are not contraindicated with E supplementation. As an aside, avoid iron if you do not need to take it because of iron-deficiency anemia. This is especially important for those of you with chronic viral infections such as hepatitis C, herpes, or chronic fatigue syndrome, or if you always catch whatever flu is going around. Iron is proviral, which means it feeds the virus. Extra iron can also make arthritis worse. Look for an iron-free multivitamin if you use one and don't need iron.

Occasionally people need to take a blood thinner, and some reports indicate that vitamin E can cause further blood thinning. More recent studies have proven that it is safe to supplement with vitamin E even when taking a very potent blood thinner such as coumadin (Warfarin). However, it would be a good precaution to stop vitamin E supplementation a few days before a sched-uled surgery. Actually, more than being a blood thinner, vitamin E causes platelets (the cells in your blood that cause scabs to form over a wound) to be less sticky. This is largely how vitamin E works to protect your heart—it pre-vents sticky platelets from building up inside the arteries and contributing to atherosclerotic plaque (narrowing of the arteries).

15.

How to Protect Your Liver

*I*n naturopathic medical school we learned again and again, "When in doubt, treat the liver." What our teachers were telling us is that the liver is the single most important organ in our bodies for detoxification, and that most human suffering is related in some degree to improper liver function. The liver has many roles in maintaining our good health, including detoxification of the thousands of chemicals we are exposed to over a lifetime. The chemical burden in our environment is likely to increase. Hopefully, cleaner energy sources and stricter controls on pesticides and industrial solvent use will provide for a cleaner environment for our great-great grandchildren, but meanwhile the number-one reason the "war on cancer" has not succeeded is environmental pollution. In addition to chemical exposure, drugs of all kinds and excess consumption of simple carbohydrates, as well as alcohol, nicotine, and saturated dietary fat, all harm the liver.

We need our liver in tip-top condition to handle current conditions. For women in any phase of menopause, excellent liver health is increasingly important as our hormonal function changes and our organs begin to age. Many popular drugs have a profoundly negative impact on our livers, including cholesterol-lowering drugs and weight-loss drugs. Always look for a natural solution to health problems before resorting to prescription drugs. Don't forget that prescription drug use is the fourth leading cause of death in the United States. Liver disease of various types falls within the top ten causes of death. Some of the general symptoms of a stressed liver include bloating, constipation, decreased fertility, fatigue, gas, hormonal irregularities, nausea, poor appetite, weakness, weight loss or gain, yellowish or itchy skin, and varicose veins, including hemorrhoids. Hormonal problems occur with a poorly functioning liver because that is where hormones are assembled and then broken down for excretion. Also, any kind of hormonal supplementation (such as HRT, progesterone cream, and the pill) will reduce bile production and flow through the liver, thus compromising liver health.

An Introduction to Bile

Bile production is one of the most important jobs of the liver. Bile is so important that the liver stores a backup supply in a special little sack, the gallbladder, which hangs underneath it. Bile is mostly made up of recycled red blood cells and enzymes, which very effectively break down dietary fat into essential fatty acids that can be used by our bodies. These essential fatty acids are absorbed into the bloodstream through the small intestine. Besides turning fat into fuel and new cell walls, bile also stimulates peristalsis in the large intestine. Peristalsis is the rhythmic movement of the large intestine (also called the colon), which promotes proper bowel evacuation. Without proper liver function people are likely to become constipated, because they don't have enough bile to flow into the gut and promote a complete bowel movement. Do not underestimate the importance of good bowel function to your health (not to speak of the satisfaction of having regular evacuations).

The gallbladder helps by providing that extra reservoir of bile needed when a fatty meal comes along and requires instant attention. It is so energy expensive to produce bile that our bodies recycle nearly 100 percent of the bile that the liver produces. The tiny bit that escapes gives the dark brown color to the stool. Keep your gallbladder if you can—it comes in handy in maintaining optimal liver health. If you are having gallbladder attacks and your doctor is recommending surgical removal, try the liver-cleansing techniques described below before removing this important little organ forever.

Beets and Other Foods to Heal Your Liver

Besides avoiding all toxins, my three favorite tools for improving liver function are beets, milk thistle, and castor oil packs. Let's start with beets, since I always like to start with the diet in making any positive health changes. Try to seek out organically grown beets, since beets are a root crop, and like carrots, are particularly prone to absorbing toxins in the soil. Beets improve liver function largely by thinning the bile, allowing it to flow more freely through the liver and into the small intestine, where it breaks down the fat and stimulates peristalsis. Another benefit of enhanced bile flow is the reduced likelihood of forming gallstones, a leading cause for surgical removal of the gallbladder. In fact, beets are one of my main therapeutic medicines for preventing and reducing the pain of gallbladder attacks.

My favorite way to prepare beets is to steam them whole, in a steamer or a pot with a small amount of water, until a fork easily pierces into the flesh. The skins should slip off quite easily when the beets are cool. Your hands will get stained in the process, but that's OK because you absorb some of the beet through your hands and it'll wash off. (Beet tops have been used as a vegetable dye since antiquity, and they produce a slightly pink, cream color.) Once the skins are removed you can cut the beets into bite-sized cubes and place them in a mason jar, where they will keep for at least a week in the fridge. I like to drizzle flax oil and balsamic vinegar over my beets to create a light pickling dressing. Serve two to four mouthfuls every other day: it's good for the whole family. Other foods containing liver-cleansing factors include the high-sulfur foods eggs, garlic, and onions; high-fiber foods, such as apples, celery, legumes, oat bran, and pears; cabbage family foods, such as bok choy, broccoli, and Brussels sprouts; and the spices cinnamon, licorice, and turmeric.

Milk Thistle

Milk thistle, *Silybum marianum,* is a well-known herbal liver protector against such major insults as carbon tetrachloride, mushroom poisoning, radiation, and Tylenol overdose. Milk thistle has been used medicinally for more than 2,000 years and has been rigorously studied for more than thirty years. An Internet search will produce hundreds of references regarding the good effects of this herb on the liver. Milk thistle helps the liver in three distinct ways. First, the active ingredient, silymarin, can incorporate itself into the liver cells and prevent the uptake of toxins into the cells by providing specific ingredients. Second, milk thistle is a potent antioxidant and prevents oxidative damage in the liver tissue. Third, milk thistle actually helps repair damaged liver cells. I instruct all of my patients with hepatitis C, or other types of hepatitis, or with a history of alcoholism, to take milk thistle. It is the most widely used botanical medicine in Russia, where alcoholism is rampant. For serious liver problems, a standardized extract of milk thistle (70 percent silymarin) should be used, 200 mg three times daily. Very few, if any, side effects are noted with milk-thistle. Since it improves bile flow it sometimes results in loose stools, but this is usually a temporary problem. Even lower doses can be effective if you are in the perimenopausal phase of menopause, especially if you have a history of using the pill or are prone to constipation but otherwise healthy. I would suggest 200 mg daily, three times a week, to help keep your liver working properly as you transition through hormonal changes. If you take in more than ten ounces of alcohol weekly, consider cutting back, or use these liver-cleansing methods more regularly. I particularly like the phytosome form of milk thistle, which is a special packaging of the milk thistle formulated to enhance its uptake into the cells.

Castor Oil

My very favorite liver-enhancing naturopathic remedy is the castor oil pack. Traditionally, castor oil has been used for a wide variety of ailments including arthritis, breast cancer, colitis, constipation, epilepsy, fibrocystic breasts, headaches, hemorrhoids, hepatitis, kidney stones, lymphedema, pelvic inflammatory disease, poisoning, and ulcers. When taken internally castor oil, also known as palma Christi (the hand of Christ) or wonder-tree, is very laxative and can also induce labor in a pregnant woman near term. An appropriate medicinal use for improving liver function is to apply castor oil *externally* over the liver and then cover the area with heat, which drives the healing oil into the skin. Numerous research studies have described the positive effect that topical castor oil has on the immune system (it increases the production of white blood cells) and the lymphatic system (it stimulates the drainage of toxins into the lymph nodes and channels). The lymphatic system is the human body's garbage collection system, picking up toxins from the blood and tissues and channeling them into the kidneys and intestines for elimination.

The old-fashioned way of using castor oil packs to stimulate drainage of congested tissues was to soak a flannel cloth with the oil, heat it in the oven, and place the warm, oily flannel over the affected area. I much prefer to use a castor-oil roll-on dispenser and then cover the area with a clean cloth. Place a heating pad on top of this for at least twenty minutes, but preferably for an hour. For a castor oil pack to the liver, apply a fairly thick layer of castor oil dispensed from the roll-on (like a deodorant stick), under the right ribcage, across the midline, and between the lower ribs on the right, including around the side of your waist. This is approximately the area under which the liver is found. The cloth is put down next, to protect the heating pad from the slightly sticky layer of castor oil and to absorb toxins drawn out through the skin. The heating pad can be held in place by a large towel pinned with a safety pin, but this is optional. I often instruct patients to apply this soothing remedy every night for a week, then several times a week thereafter for several months.

I ask all my hepatitis patients to use castor oil packs regularly to improve their liver function. Even if you don't have a liver disease, your liver is largely responsible for the symptoms of hormonal changes, in which case you will benefit from this method of enhancing your liver function. If you have fibro-cystic breasts that get especially tender premenstrually, apply the castor oil pack to your breasts daily at the first indication of increased tenderness. Consult a doctor if your breast pain is new, sudden, or in one breast only. If you tend to constipation, drink more water, increase the fiber in your diet, and apply castor oil packs regularly to your abdomen.

I usually recommend that castor oil packs be applied at night, and simply left in place overnight, but always turn off the heating pad before you fall asleep. If necessary, the skin may be cleansed with baking soda diluted by plenty of water after using a castor oil pack. Dip a cloth into the soda water and rub the skin briskly until it is no longer sticky. Usually the oil soaks in completely within an hour, and no cleaning is needed.

Castor oil is also a wonderful first-aid remedy for bruises, fractures, sprains, and strains. Applied topically, with or without heat, it greatly reduces the pain, swelling, and bruising caused by a soft-tissue injury to any part of the body. Apply castor oil directly to the affected area and continue treatment for up to forty-eight hours, applying more oil as it is absorbed by the body. Castor oil also works well for chapped lips, to lighten dark patches on the skin (liver spots), and to relieve the irritation of insect bites. For castor oil roll-ons and more information about this marvelous natural substance, you can contact Gen MacManiman, in Fall City, Washington at 1-425-222-5587.

16.

Phytoestrogens

*P*hyto is the Greek word for plant; phytoestrogens are plant compounds that act like estrogens in the body. Along with progesterone, estrogen is what creates the menstrual cycle. Unlike progesterone, estrogen continues to be secreted throughout life, even beyond the cessation of menses. There is a slow decline of all the hormones in the years before the actual menopause, with progesterone waning first. Fewer and fewer of our menstrual cycles are ovulatory (where the dropping of an egg occurs) as we age, and without ovulation no progesterone is secreted from the ovaries. Just before we stop menstruating for good at the very end of perimenopause our estrogen supply starts to drop off and continues to do so over the next three to five years. Until menopause is established, however, many women may actually be in a state of relative estrogen dominance and have more estrogen relative to progesterone compared to before the onset of perimenopause. Progesterone is rapidly waning, but the estrogen supply remains constant, so the proportion of estrogen to progesterone is *relatively* higher than before. This can create problems typical of high-estrogen levels, including aggressive feelings, anxiety, heavier menstrual bleeding, hot flashes, night sweats, periodic headaches, sleep disturbances, tender breasts, uterine fibroid growth, water retention, and weight gain. One solution for women during this phase is to supplement with progesterone to restore the optimal ratio between progesterone and estrogen. If this route is chosen be sure it is progesterone, *not* progestin or any of the patented versions of progesterone, because none of those are exactly identical to human progesterone. It is also not wild yam cream, unless the cream contains a verifiable amount of USP progesterone.

However, this chapter is about plant estrogens, or phytoestrogens. You may be wondering why you'd use plant estrogens if you want to *reduce* the estrogen to progesterone ratio. Part of the answer is because phytoestrogens don't behave like our own estrogen in the human body. When our own estrogen comes into contact with a cell receptor, a series of reactions is initiated that stimulate the genetic information inside that cell. The cell receptor is like an antenna, very specific to particular substances, sticking out of the cell surface. Sometimes the cell receptor is described as a lock for which there is a particular key. Only that key will open the door, or turn on the genetic information. In this discussion estrogen is the key that fits into the lock of the cell receptor, and this estrogen key stimulates the genes programmed to respond to estrogen in the nucleus (center) of the cell. All of the 6 billion or so cells in the human body work this way. When human estrogen is the key in the lock, this gene stimulation forms new protein which turns on all of estrogen's effects (skin elasticity, uterine lining growth, vaginal lubrication, water retention, and so on). By contrast, when plant estrogen is the key this chain reaction is blocked, not initiated. Instead of stimulating the genetic information in the nucleus of the cell, the plant estrogen key sits in the lock but doesn't open it, and doesn't turn on the genetic information in the cell. Phytoestrogens actually *reduce* estrogen-type reactions by blocking the keyholes in the cells and lessening the interaction of cells with circulating human estrogen.

Berries, cereals, flaxseed, fruits, nuts, soybeans, several herbs (mostly black cohosh and red clover), and teas are all sources of plant estrogens. Burdock root, dong quai root (*Angelica sinensis*), licorice root, and Mexican wild yam root also contain phytoestrogens.

Soy (Glycine maximus)

Soybeans are considered the most potent food source of phytoestrogens. Not only does soy bind the most tightly to estrogen receptors on cells, but soy also binds to circulating human estrogen, thus lowering the blood levels of active estrogen. The active component of the soybean that binds to estrogen receptors is a group of plant substances called isoflavones. About 50 mg daily of soy isoflavones (about one cup of soy milk or one-half cup of soy nuts) is sufficient to offset the pesky problems caused by excess estrogen if you are in the perimenopausal phase. I particularly like a warm miso soup with chunks of firm soy tofu, carrots, garlic, ginger, onions, and plenty of kelp or dulce. Miso is a soybean paste widely available in health food and grocery stores. Soy nuts are a tasty, crunchy snack and probably pack more phytoestrogen content than any other form of soy (except powdered concentrates). Edamame, fresh soybeans, are delicious as a snack, or in soups. You may also enjoy marinated tofu, which are blocks of soybean curd soaked in delicious seasonings. Tofu alone doesn't have much taste, but it is a handy meat substitute for stir-fries or pasta sauces.

Soy and Heart Health

Several studies have proven that women using soy products had significantly fewer hot flashes than women not using soy. Soy products are often mixed with bone-building nutrients (such as calcium and vitamin D), so regular consumption of soy products can help maintain strong, healthy bones. Soy protein supplements (such as powders) have been shown to consistently lower bad LDL cholesterol without lowering the good HDL cholesterol in perimenopausal women. This is important because total cholesterol production often rises as our hormones change and the liver has more work keeping up with hormonal fluctuations. Do not be bamboozled into taking a cholesterol-lowering drug because your total cholesterol creeps up to 235 or so during this time of hormonal transition. (See Chapter 21 for more information on cholesterol testing.) Statins, the most popular class of cholesterol-lowering medication, have been shown to cause cancer in lab rats, and they also notoriously deplete Coenzyme Q_{10}, a supernutrient which promotes healthy heart function, and which tends to decline with age. If you must take a statin drug, also supplement with CoQ_{10}, 30–100 mg daily. On the subject of heart health, note that while men suffer from fatty deposits and inflammation in the arteries (arteriosclerosis), women get heart attacks because of cramps in the heart vessels. Premature cardiovascular death in women is usually completely different from cardiovascular death in men. There are two very important aspects to this information. First, unlike men, slightly elevated cholesterol levels in women approaching menopause is *normal,* and should not be medicated. Stay away from animal fats, but don't use drugs. Second, plant estrogens, such as the soy isoflavones, can not only help lower bad cholesterol, but have also been shown to improve the elasticity of the arteries, making them less prone to cramping. Women's heart attacks are more likely to be caused by cramping of the heart muscle, whereas men have heart attacks because of atherosclerosis, which reduces oxygen flow to the heart and brain. (Magnesium, my favorite smooth-muscle relaxant, is also useful for any kind of cramps, including heart vessel, leg, and menstrual.)

Soy Caveats

Although soy can offer significant benefits to perimenopausal women, there are some important issues to be aware of when using soy supplementation. Soy is such a powerful source of phytoestrogen there is concern that it may adversely affect women with certain conditions or a family history or susceptibility to estrogen-related diseases.

Thyroid Problems

First, soy is not the best choice to relieve perimenopausal symptoms if you have low thyroid function, because soy blocks thyroid receptors as well as estrogen receptors. Excess soy consumption can actually reduce thyroid function, leading to constipation, hair loss, lethargy, and lowered body temperature. In Japan, soy products are traditionally served with high-iodine foods such as sea vegetables because thyroid hormones are made from iodine. It would be a good idea for us to follow the traditional Asian habit of eating soy with seaweed for this reason. Be aware of your thyroid function before embarking on a tofu kick. At the very least, check your TSH level if you have doubts about your thyroid. (See Chapter 19 to learn more about how to check for thyroid changes.)

Genetically Modified Organisms

The second, very important, caveat about soy consumption is to avoid—no, *boycott*—genetically modified soy. By now almost everyone will have at least heard of GMO (genetically modified organisms) food. Soy, corn, and canola oil are the most widely distributed GMO foods. The idea of GMO food makes me very nervous. Europe refuses to import GMO corn and soy from the United States, causing a glut on the world market. Even starving countries in Africa are refusing to accept donations of GMO corn and soy. This is not only because the African leaders are concerned about the impact of GMO food on their people, but also because they don't want GMO seed stock to infiltrate their crops. While proponents of GMO claim that crops manipulated to be more pest resistant, or larger, or more uniform, and will allow for greater food stores to feed the world, be advised that this is an unregulated experiment with human health. It is not out of the question that GMO experiments could breed new, disease-causing viruses that cannot be controlled. I urge you to read labels and *only* purchase soy, corn, and canola-oil containing products that are certified organic, because that precludes GMO. If the soy or corn product is not organic, you can almost be guaranteed it is GMO. The bottom line is that the megacorporations like Monsanto and Nestlé stand to profit from GMO. The average consumer stands to lose. I often wonder why the executives of these corporations are not more concerned about the health and well-being of their children, grandchildren and great grandchildren. I certainly am, and no GMO food is served in our house.

I recently read "Rogue Corn on the Loose," a fascinating article published in *World Watch,* which documents the hazards of GMO corn and the fact that most of the world, besides the United States, seems aware of the risks of GMO crops. A traditional farmer in Mexico was asked how valuable he considers his heritage seed stock, how concerned he was about contamination of his seed by GMO crops, and the importance he placed on maintaining the genetically diverse seed stock he had inherited from the previous generations of farmers in his family. His answer was clear: "A handful of my seed is worth more to me than my large old stone walled family home. An earthquake could destroy my home, but my corn seed inherited from my grandparents can be planted by a hundred future generations of my descendants, to yield healthy vigorous crops." Because GMO crops are stronger (more pest and disease resistant) than pure stock, GMO crops could ultimately destroy the diversity and availability of natural crops. Avoid GMO food, and be aware that products containing canola oil, corn, and soy are almost certainly GMO if they are not labeled as certified organic. We as consumers can wield huge political (financial) power, so let's nip the GMO disaster in the bud.

Flaxseed (*Linum usitatissimum*)

After soybeans, flaxseeds are the next highest food source of phytoestrogens. Flaxseeds are also very high in cancer-preventing compounds known as lignans, plant substances that get broken down by beneficial intestinal bacteria and then circulate through the liver. In the liver, the lignans modulate the production, availability, and action of the hormones produced in our bodies. Studies have shown that women who consume ground-up flaxseeds, or flaxseed oil, have lowered levels of estrogen (especially the potentially cancer-causing E2), similar to the effects seen with soy isoflavones.

Flax Oil Is a Good Fat

The best dietary fats are flax oil, coconut oil, fish oils, and olive oil. Besides containing lots of phytoestrogens, the good thing about flaxseed is that it is the only plant source of an essential fat, omega-3 essential fatty acid. Essential fats, like the essential amino acids, cannot be produced in the body and must be consumed. Good-quality fats are critical for blood vessel, brain, heart, and skin health. In fact, every single one of our 6 billion cells is surrounded by a double fat layer that protects the nucleus and tiny organs within the cell. The quality of the fats in our diet determines the quality (flexibility and durability) of all the cells in our bodies. Fats and oils that are solid at room temperature tend to make our cell walls stiff and dysfunctional. The omega-3 fats allow for a strong, yet flexible cell membrane.

Although coconut oil is a saturated fat, it is a reasonable choice for stir-frying if used sparingly because it is more stable at higher heats than most fats, it is not hydrogenated, and it has no trans-fatty acids. It consists of 50 percent lauric acid, a good fat, and structurally is a medium chain triglyceride, which the body can metabolize efficiently and convert into energy rather than store as fat. Fish oils are high in the beneficial omega-3 fats, which not only keep the cells (including our skin) flexible and functional, but also reverse the damage caused by inflammation of any kind. For example, omega-3 oils are highly beneficial for such inflammatory conditions as allergic responses, asthma, chronic hives, and rheumatoid arthritis.

As mentioned above, flax is particularly valuable as the only plant that is high in these omega-3 fats. All other sources that are high in omega-3 oils are animal products. I used to dispense prescriptions for one to three table-spoons of flaxseed oil daily to most of my patients, but I have converted to prescribing freshly ground flaxseeds because the oil they release is so fresh and the ground seeds provide much-needed extra fiber.

Try to avoid saturated fats, and especially hydrogenated fats like margarine and Crisco. Poor quality fats are often used in commercially available baked goods, in salad dressings, and certainly in fried foods. Deep fried is the worst way to consume fats because the oils have been degraded by high heat, and once in our bodies, they will proceed to degrade our blood vessels, brain, and skin.

Flaxseeds Reduce Breast-Cancer Risk

It is widely accepted that estrogen promotes most breast cancers. Women with a long history of using the pill and women using hormone replacement therapy are all at higher risk for breast cancer. Several studies have shown that regular ingestion of flaxseeds will lower the estrogen that promotes tumor growth in the breasts. This alone should be a good enough reason for anyone with breasts to regularly consume flaxseeds.

How to Use Flaxseeds in Your Diet

I recommend supplementing your diet with three tablespoons of freshly ground flaxseeds, three to seven times weekly, stirred into juice or water. It's a delicious, thick drink that not only provides extremely fresh omega-3 oils, but also is an effective source of bulking fiber. You'll need a little coffee-bean-type electric grinder, because your molars won't quite do the trick for breaking open the hard shell covering the flaxseed. You can use ground flaxseeds on your morning oatmeal, stir them into yogurt, sprinkle them on salads, or bake them into muffins (baked goods tend to brown more quickly with flaxseed meal in the recipe). You can also cut down on the oil called for in baked goods by substituting flax meal. If a recipe requires one-third cup of oil, replace it with one cup of flaxseed meal. Grind it yourself to ensure that the delicate oils are as fresh as possible. Of the two varieties available, the golden flaxseeds are thought to have a higher omega-3 oil content (the darker seeds are also used for commercial linseed oil).

It is very important to keep the colon clean and without regular elimination, we quickly become toxic, so this high-quality fiber will help most people to have regular bowel movements.

Black Cohosh (*Cimicifuga racemosa*)

In Germany, the most widely studied phytoestrogenic herbal medicine is undoubtedly black cohosh (not to be confused with blue cohosh, a very strong uterine stimulant that can cause miscarriages). In studies comparing black cohosh to horse-estrogen (Premarin) use in perimenopausal women, the plant medicine had favorable effects on bone and cholesterol, and no harmful effect on the uterus (unlike Premarin, which can cause endometrial cancer). This is different than soy, which helps with high-estrogen problems like hot flashes, but has not been shown to help with preventing osteoporosis unless it is mixed with other bone builders. The isoflavones in black cohosh are somewhat different than those in soy or flax.

Black cohosh may be the single most effective plant remedy for controlling hot flashes. I use it regularly, with good success, for my perimenopausal and menopausal patients. The usual dose is to start with 20 mg of standardized black cohosh twice daily. This can be increased to 200 mg twice daily, if needed, with no unwanted side effects. Black cohosh is currently marketed (expensively) by a drug company as Remifemin, but you can find equivalent good-quality black cohosh supplements in most health food stores.

Lydia Pinkham's Ladies' Powder

About 150 years ago, an enterprising woman named Lydia Pinkham brought her home pharmacy and knowledge of plant medicine from England to the new world, America. This pioneer is said to have traveled on covered wagons across the country to California and Alaska, selling her wares and teaching women about home remedies. By far her most popular product, Lydia Pinkham's Ladies' Powder was simply pure black cohosh root, ground and ready to be mixed into warm water for drinking.

Red Clover (*Trifolium pratense*)

Red clover extract (marketed as Promensil) has also been shown to relieve hot flashes, although not as dramatically as black cohosh or soy. My experience with red clover is that it can worsen breast tenderness, so I rarely choose this herb for treating hormonal problems, but I include it here as an option for those who do not have a problem with breast tenderness.

PART THREE

Where Hormones Come From

17.

The Adrenal Glands

You have probably heard of adrenaline in the context of something scary giving you a shot or burst of adrenaline. Maybe you've read a magazine article about high-adrenaline sports (like sky diving). Adrenaline, also known as epinephrine, is not just a turn of phrase; it is a very real secretion from the adrenal glands. The term adrenaline comes from the Latin root words *ad* (above) and *renal* (kidney); and epinephrine is from the Greek root words *epi* (above) and *nephron* (kidney). Both names are anatomically descriptive. The adrenal glands sit right above the kidneys, which are protected by the lower back ribcage. The action of adrenaline is to shunt blood away from the digestive tract and skin, and toward the brain, heart, leg muscles, and lungs. In other words, a shot of adrenaline prepares us for fight or flight.

Back when our survival depended on being able to hunt, run fast, and protect ourselves and our families, adrenaline rushes literally saved our lives. This fight-or-flight mode is deeply ingrained in human behavior. These days, we don't normally encounter threats to our lives on a regular basis, but we do regularly encounter chronic stressors, such as bills, people we don't get along with, bad news, and chronic pain such as arthritis. All these stressors make us less hearty, and more susceptible to illness. Chronic stress causes unnecessary chronic adrenaline secretion from the adrenal glands, which can lead to bone loss, deterioration of skin quality, digestive upsets, inflammation of all kinds, poor immune health, and ultimately, cancer. The best way to control chronic stress is by methodically removing unnecessary stressors and purposefully pursuing calming activities such as deep breathing, meditation, nature walks, warm water soaks, and yoga.

If we approach transitions like the one into menopause with good cheer and calm, we are much less likely to burn out and age quickly.

Not Just Adrenaline: The Role of DHEA

Adrenaline cannot be measured in the body because it only lasts for about a minute in the bloodstream after being secreted. The adrenal glands don't just secrete adrenaline, though; they also secrete DHEA, cortisol, and aldosterone. Let's start with DHEA (dehydroepiandrosterone), which is the most abundant hormone in the body. All hormones derive from cholesterol, and most of the cholesterol in the body turns into DHEA. DHEA can then convert, on demand, to progesterone, estrogen, and testosterone. As we age, and as women approach menopause, it is normal for cholesterol levels to rise slightly in response to waning hormone levels. All our glands secrete lower amounts of hormones as we age, not just the ovaries. As the levels of DHEA decline, cholesterol often rises in an attempt to provide more building blocks for new hormone formation.

Cortisol

The adrenal glands also secrete cortisol, the body's natural anti-inflammatory substance. If we are chronically stressed and chronically secreting adrenaline, DHEA, and cortisol, these substances will be wasted and our reserves will run low. This is why chronic stress can lead to all types of inflammation, such as joints that ache, lower back pain, pain after eating, and stuffy nose. Unlike adrenaline, cortisol lingers in the bloodstream for a while, and can be used to measure adrenal function. Cortisol levels can point the doctor toward understanding your overall adrenal health. (By studying the cortisol molecule, pharmacists and biochemists were able to create synthetic versions, such as the drugs cortisone and prednisone, which became the big-guns therapy for many doctors trying to control inflammation and swelling.) Ultimately, cortisol is suppressive to the immune system.

Cortisol travels around the blood attached to a sugar molecule and actually doubles as blood sugar overnight, when we are not eating. Thus, cortisol should be at its high point (but not too high) first thing in the morning. As soon as we put food into our mouths, cortisol levels should go down and continue to drop toward the low daily levels at bedtime. In overstressed people, however, cortisol levels may stay high all day. This means the person is putting out adrenaline (and all the other adrenal secretions) all day long. I find the saliva cortisol tests particularly useful for evaluating adrenal function in my patients. Four saliva samples are collected during a twenty-four hour period, and sent to a lab for analysis. The original Adrenal Stress Index saliva test was created by Dr. Elias Ilya, medical director of Diagnos-Techs, Inc., a clinical and research lab in the Seattle, Washington area. Conventional doctors tend to evaluate adrenal function with a more invasive test that involves injections and a series of blood draws.

What Fatigue Does to Your Body

Some of the signs of poor adrenal function are weight gain around the middle (the most dangerous in terms of heart health), bone loss, and sugar cravings. Other signs include hypoglycemia, increased allergic reactions, a moon-shaped face, or a buffalo hump developing at the base of the neck. Before these changes occur, however, there will be low energy, low sex drive, migraines, muscle and joint pain, poor memory, and poor sleep.

The body typically heals at night. Skin regeneration, for example, occurs mostly during sleep. If we are chronically stressed, however, and adrenal output is constantly being triggered, the continually high cortisol levels will interfere with optimal nighttime skin regeneration and all other healing.

Adrenal Tonics

The best way to approach adrenal repair is rest. Get your eight hours of sleep; don't skimp. Identify and avoid stressors if possible. Stay well hydrated. In addition to these simple steps, a number of natural supplements are available to help build adrenal gland function.

Vitamin C

Vitamin C is a specific nutrient for the adrenal gland because these small, immensely powerful glands have the highest content of vitamin C per gram of any other tissue in the body. You can take lots of vitamin C—to bowel tolerance—because vitamin C is water-soluble and you cannot overdose on it. However, you can only absorb about 4 grams (4,000 mg) at a time (most people get far less than 4 grams of vitamin C daily). I like drinking powdered, buffered vitamin C because that helps me get enough water, too. ("Buffered" means the acidity of the vitamin C is balanced with minerals so it is ready for absorption into the blood and tissues. "To bowel tolerance" means until your stools become loose.)

Case Study: Adrenal Fatigue

Suzanne, a pleasant thirty-four-year-old woman with regular, light-flow menses, came to my office because of chronic dizziness. She told me that she used to be very active in the community, but in the past year had been forced to curtail her activity beyond work and the domestic basics. She said she would often miss the curb or a step, and described feeling as though she could easily black out. She preferred to walk with a friend who could provide a steadying arm.

Her favorite brother, his wife, and their two children had been in a fatal car accident eighteen months before. Her mother had died "of grief" just a few months prior to Suzanne's visit to me. Her hair was thinning and she had lost weight due to a reduced appetite. Her worst new problem was migraines, much worse premenstrually and at ovulation.

A physical exam revealed normal blood pressure, heart sounds, pulse, reflexes, and temperature. She was thin, with dark circles under her eyes. She had a mild tenderness on either side of the spine in the midback, site of the adrenal glands, and her pupils did not respond appropriately to light stimulation. (Normally, when a doctor shines a little penlight into your eyes, the pupils constrict and stay tight under the glare of the light. In people who have adrenal fatigue though, as Suzanne did, the pupils will initially constrict, but then dilate again despite the ongoing burden of light.) The four-sample saliva test confirmed chronically high cortisol and very low DHEA levels, so I began supplementation with 25 mg of DHEA daily, and 2 grams a day of licorice in a solid extract form (sorry, the candy twists just won't do).

Within two weeks, Suzanne said she was sleeping better, had gained several pounds, and no longer felt subject to fainting (her aldosterone was working better to keep her blood pressure normal). After another month, Suzanne reported that she no longer needed to lean on her husband while walking, and she was exploring community service work with Hospice (an organization to facilitate dying at home with dignity).

B Vitamins

The B vitamins are known to be antistress vitamins because they provide direct nutrition to the nervous system. Vitamin B_5 (pantothenic acid) is particularly helpful in reducing adrenal fatigue. Nicotine and caffeine whip up the adrenal glands, inappropriately creating the fight-or-flight response, and B5, along with the other Bs, can help mitigate this unnecessary adrenaline response. Quitting nicotine and caffeine works even better, needless to say.

DHEA

If DHEA is low, supplementation will help to restore adrenal health. In general, women should not take more than 25 mg of DHEA daily, and men should limit their intake to 50 mg daily. Higher doses are probably fine short term. Biotin (a B vitamin) and the trace mineral zinc are both catalysts in DHEA formation, and may be all you need to promote adequate DHEA levels. Weightlifting will also stimulate DHEA production without taxing the adrenal glands. Work with a trainer for at least one or two sessions to figure out a good routine before setting off on your own.

Licorice

Licorice (*Glycyrrhiza glabra*) is one of my favorite adrenal tonics. It can raise the blood pressure of those who are prone to hypertension by stimulating urinary excretion of potassium. If high blood pressure is not a problem for you, licorice is a perfect remedy for stress, especially if your stress is held in the stomach and digestive tract. Use up to 2 grams daily with food. If you do have high blood pressure, look for the DGL form of licorice or make sure to take a potassium supplement daily (99 mg).

18.
The Ovaries

Researcher and breast surgeon Dr. Susan Love likes to quip that menopause is "puberty in reverse!" She's got a point; as a girl's ovaries mature, her breasts and pubic hair emerge, and then, within a few years, she starts menstruation with all the accompanying hormonal mood fluctuations. Skipping ahead forty or so years, the ovaries begin to fade until their secretions can no longer create a menstrual cycle, and again many of us experience a few roller-coaster years.

The ovaries are actually two egg sacs located near the top of the uterus that are attached to the uterus by the fallopian tubes. The ovaries fill two major functions: reproduction (they contain eggs), and the secretion of sex hormones, which cause breasts to grow and menstrual cycles to occur. Each ovary resembles a small almond. The non-pregnant uterus is a fairly small organ, about the size and shape of an upside-down pear. The uterus and ovaries are protected in front by the pubic bone and in the back by the sacrum (sacred bone) that is formed by the five fused vertebrae at the base of the spine. The female embryo within the womb of a pregnant woman holds nearly 4 million eggs in her tiny ovaries. (My mom got a big smile on her face when she realized that the egg that became my daughter, her granddaughter, had once been contained in her own uterus.) By the time a baby girl is one year old, she has only 1 million or so viable eggs remaining. By the end of a woman's menstrual cycling (median age fifty-one), only a few thousand eggs remain at most. The ovaries shrink at menopause as their secretions diminish, and can seldom, if ever, be felt by a doctor giving a pelvic exam. Palpable ovaries in postmenopausal women require further investigation.

Menstruation Is Lunar

Our hormonal cycles typically follow the waxing and waning of the moon. Since the dawn of civilization, women have associated themselves with the moon. The word menses is derived from the same root word as moon. When tribes of women lived close to the earth, with a clean diet and without artificial light, they would menstruate at the same time, usually at the full moon. In the part of the world now known as the Middle East, "menstruating" women would gather together in red tents to arrange marriages, inventory the food supplies, and plan the activities of the tribe for the next month. During the forty or so years that women menstruate, the lunar cycling persists if the ovaries are healthy.

At ovulation each month, the fertile woman will drop one egg, usually alternating between the right and left ovaries. After ovulation, the egg only stays alive for a day maximum, although sperm can live up to five days in the vagina or uterus. This should be of interest to couples practicing natural birth control, or for timing pregnancies, since a woman can only conceive in the twenty-four hours following the one-day ovulation period. The egg carries only the X-shaped sex chromosome, and thus is female. The sperm carries either the X or the Y chromosome, which is why the male partner is responsible for the sex of the fetus. Chromosomally speaking, the male sex is XY, whereas the female sex is XX.

Healthy Ovaries Are Yellow

In my cadaver anatomy class at medical school, I remember being very impressed by the vivid yellow color of the ovaries of a young, healthy woman who had died in an accident. Healthy ovaries are chock-full of beta-carotene, the water-soluble precursor to vitamin A, which is naturally deep orange to bright yellow in color. The ripened follicle that contains the egg bursting out of the ovarian sac at ovulation is called the *corpus luteum,* or yellow body. This was very valuable information because, in my clinical practice, I have helped several previously infertile women achieve pregnancy simply by supplementing them with beta-carotene.

The Follicular Phase

The first half of the menstrual cycle, which starts with day one of the menstrual period, when the endometrium is shed, is called the follicular phase, because the ovaries are filled with developing follicles (which protect the immature eggs). The follicular phase lasts about fourteen days, and culminates in ovulation in the mid-point of the monthly cycle. As we approach meno-pause the follicular phase may become quite variable because there are fewer eggs left in the ovaries toward the end of our childbearing years and therefore fewer ovulations. If the follicular phase is shortened, it is quite typical in per-imenopause to have shortened menstrual cycles, so although you may have had a twenty-nine day cycle for twenty years, in your late thirties or early forties your cycle might shorten to twenty-five, twenty-three, or even twenty-one days.

The Luteal Phase

The second half of the cycle, from ovulation until the next menstrual period, is called the luteal phase and is characterized by rising progesterone levels. If no pregnancy occurs in this half of the cycle, the progesterone levels decline quickly, signaling the go-ahead for the uterus to shed its endometrial lining at the beginning of the next menstrual cycle. This shedding of the endometrium is menstruation (frequently called having a period), which occurs at the begin-ning of the next follicular phase. The luteal phase tends to stay fairly constant, between twelve to sixteen days. The luteal phase hormone, progesterone (mean-ing "for gestation"), is the first hormone to wane as we approach menopause, declining as we have fewer ovulations. Next, in perimenopause, estrogen lev-els decline, and finally testosterone levels decrease. Older women wishing to carry a healthy pregnancy to term can help prevent miscarriages by taking supplemental progesterone in the first trimester of their pregnancy.

All Kinds of Hormones

The ovaries secrete three major sex hormones: estrogen, progesterone, and testosterone. Women generate a respectable amount of the so-called male hor-mone, testosterone, and continue to do so even after menopause. The female sex hormones (estrogen and progesterone) are secreted according to where you are in your monthly cycle, but testosterone is steadily secreted every day. Many tissues in the body have hormone receptors (brain, bones, gut, and sex organs) which receive the sex hormones in a cyclic fashion. It is important to keep the cyclical nature of hormonal secretion in mind when attempting hor-mone replacement of the female hormones, and to understand that it doesn't make sense to take the same amount of estrogen and progesterone every day, particularly during perimenopause. The release of these hormones from the ovaries is directed by the pituitary (a master gland in the brain) in response to feedback from blood and tissue.

Although many variations of estrogen exist, we are principally concerned with estrone (E1) and estradiol (E2), which together comprise 10 to 20 percent of circulating estrogens, and estriol (E3), which is weaker and makes up to 90 percent of circulating estrogens, as discussed in Chapter 11. Conventional hormone replacement often delivers only estradiol, which has a strong positive effect on bone, but a bad effect on breast, heart, and uterine tissue. Examples of estradiol-only drugs include Premarin (a pill), Estraderm (the patch) and Estrace (the cream). Many conventional doctors still prescribe hormone replacement therapy (HRT) containing estradiol derived from the urine of pregnant mares (hence the name of the popular drug Premarin).

Waning Hormones

The pituitary gland in the brain secretes FSH (follicular stimulating hormone) in response to waning estrogen levels, and secretes LH (luteinizing hormone) in response to waning progesterone levels. An FSH level above forty suggests that there is inadequate estrogen to ensure ovulation. Many doctors use a rise in FSH levels to confirm impending menopause, but since FSH levels may vary dramatically in the same woman on the same day, they are not a reliable indicator, particularly in a woman who is still menstruating.

The waning of all these hormones, starting with progesterone, then the various estrogens, and lastly testosterone, is the *true* indicator of the onset of menopause. Only in the last year of perimenopause (which can start as early as the mid-thirties and last up to fifteen years) do estrogen levels drop significantly. In fact, estrogen levels may actually *increase* right before menopause, which spurs the rapid growth of uterine fibroids, and breast and ovarian cysts. Eventually, estrogen levels are reduced to the point of not allowing an egg to drop (ovulation) and not producing a menstrual shedding of the endometrium from the uterus, and menopause begins. The strict definition of the start of menopause is twelve months after the last period.

Progesterone Wanes First

Lower progesterone levels are likely to be the culprit in many premenopausal symptoms, which can include some, all, or none of the following: menstrual irregularities, changes in memory and cognition, decreased libido, depression, facial acne and hair growth, fatigue, headaches, head hair loss, hot flashes, mood swings, nausea, palpitations, skin changes, sleep disturbances, urinary tract infections (the result of thinning bladder wall and urethral tissues), vaginal dryness and thinning, and the beginning stages of heart disease and osteoporosis. The increase in estrogen toward the end of the perimenopausal period may be absolute, or may be relative compared to progesterone levels. The concept of relative estrogen dominance in perimenopause has received much publicity thanks to the work of Dr. John Lee, of Sebastopol, CA. Dr. Lee has almost single-handedly created the huge demand for progesterone among the perimenopausal crowd. Many women *are* dramatically helped by supplementing with progesterone for the unpleasant symptoms of estrogen domi-

Case Study: Ovarian Cancer

Helen, an attractive, if pale, seventy-eight-year-old woman, came to see me about memory changes, urinary discomfort, and occasional incontinence. Her history revealed that her menses had briefly stopped when she was forty-eight. She went to a doctor who promptly diagnosed her as menopausal, and placed her on Prempro, a conventional hormone mix consisting of Premarin, usually 0.625 mg of equine estadiol, and Provera, a synthetic progestin, which allowed her to continue her monthly periods.

During my physical exam, I noticed that Helen had very pale mucous membranes, especially inside the lower eyelid (they should be bright red), and a five-centimeter mass in the left lower part of her abdomen, plus slightly engorged lymph nodes in her left groin area. Basic lab work confirmed that she had iron-deficiency anemia from prolonged bleeding (she was still having regular periods), and that her pelvic mass needed further workup to rule out ovarian cancer.

Amazed that she was still taking the Prempro, I stopped it immediately and begin her on a liquid iron supplement. A brief mental-status questionnaire showed that Helen was well-oriented, so I was less concerned about dementia than about a low blood supply to the brain. Although it turned out that she did have ovarian cancer, possibly stimulated by her many years of unnecessary hormone support, she recovered quite quickly from her anemia and was able to tolerate the cancer treatment. Surgery to eliminate her pelvic tumor resolved her bladder problems, and as of this writing she is alive, well, and happy at the age of eighty-seven.

Case Study: Progesterone

Caroline, a thirty-seven-year-old mother of infant twins, had conceived them after several spontaneous miscarriages. She was now concerned because she was having severe breast tenderness, was constipated and always felt abnormally full after eating, and was always very sleepy and depressed. She had used progesterone supplementation to help prevent another miscarriage during her pregnancy, and had generally felt very well throughout it.

On close questioning, Caroline revealed that she was continuing with transdermal progesterone because she thought it would help her energy and prevent post-partum depression. She said she wasn't sure it was working well even though she applied about one teaspoon or more twice daily. This is the equivalent of at least 200 mg of oral Progesterone daily, but the topical creams can be much more potent because they bypass the liver and get absorbed directly into the bloodstream. A blood check confirmed that her progesterone levels were, in fact, off the chart. I suspected this because breast tenderness, poor digestion, and sleepiness are classic signs of progesterone excess, a fairly rare condition which can occur with progesterone supplementation, particularly transdermal application.

Caroline's symptoms could easily have been attributed to being an older mom of new twins, nursing a lot, not getting much sleep, and not having time to prepare good food for herself. But luckily she was honest with me about her progesterone supplementation. Her troubling symptoms diminished and she started to feel better within just a few days of discontinuing the progesterone cream, although it took several more months to help the twins sleep through the night so mom could sleep, too.

nance such as heavy bleeding, increased food cravings, irritability, menstrual cramping, or shortened menstrual cycles, but be aware that transdermal (applied to the skin) and oral progesterone can greatly increase our progesterone levels at a time when our bodies are naturally trying to make less progesterone. So, if you elect to use supplemental progesterone, follow the instructions carefully and have your progesterone levels monitored regularly through blood or saliva tests.

Progesterone Won't Prevent Osteoporosis

Although his work on progesterone has helped women, not everything Dr. Lee claims has proven to be true. Most important is that, there is no good evidence that progesterone supplementation can prevent bone loss, although he says it can. It is well known that bone loss accelerates after menopause, which suggests that female hormones have a role in maintaining bone density. Bone loss may also be partly due to declining levels of vitamin D as we age, since vitamin D is crucial for the absorption of minerals into the bone. It is a fat-based molecule like the female hormones and is considered a pro-hormone.

In numerous clinical studies, estrogens have consistently been shown to maintain and improve bone density. One of the reasons given for supplementing estrogen at menopause is to prevent bone loss, which cannot be arrested by any other treatments. (The only other reason I might use estrogen on a patient would be to treat out-of-control hot flashes.) In menopausal women generally, the increased risk of breast, ovarian, and uterine cancer incurred by equine or synthetic estrogen use is not offset by the benefit of strong bones. There are safer, more effective, and less expensive ways to protect your bones, brain, breasts, heart, liver, and uterus.

19.

The Thyroid Gland

The thyroid gland is located just above the pit of the throat, near the surface of the neck, and it is the approximate shape and size of a bow-tie pasta noodle, perhaps a tad larger. If the pit of your throat doesn't have an olive-sized indentation, you may have a thyroid problem. The thyroid gland can be thought of as the body's gas pedal (or brake, if it isn't working). The hormones in the thyroid regulate body temperature, growth, and physical development. Broadly speaking, the thyroid determines the metabolic rate of your body, and when your thyroid gland is working properly, your blood pressure, body weight, and energy levels are stable. When it's not functioning well it can result in problems that mimic classic perimenopausal and menopausal symptoms.

In the fairly recent old days, doctors used to evaluate thyroid function with a thorough medical history and a physical exam that included taking the temperature and checking the Achilles tendon reflex. The Achilles tendon is the back of the ankle, and so called because the mother of the mythical hero Achilles dipped him into a liquid to protect him from death while holding him at the ankle, so the Achilles tendon became a metaphor for a point of vulnerability. As recently as fifty years ago a machine was used to tap a reflex hammer on the back of the Achilles tendon, and transcribe, via a pen attached to the patient's big toe, the pattern of the jerking tendon onto a roll of graph paper. The closer together the spikes were on the graph, the more active the thyroid gland. Now we can isolate the thyroid hormones as well as all the precursor chemicals that cause the thyroid to release these hormones in the blood. This gives us a more complete picture and is more precise than the Achilliometer.

In my practice, I use a brisk tap with a reflex hammer on the back of the Achilles tendon to begin the thyroid exam, but no pen taped to the toe. If the patient's reflex is blunted or absent, I'll ask, "Are you constipated?" or "Are your menstrual bleeds heavy?" because both are signs of low thyroid function. The many other common symptoms of low thyroid function include: brittle nails, depression, dizziness, dry skin, fatigue, feeling chilly, frequent infections, hair loss, high blood pressure, inability to lose weight despite calorie reduction, joint aches, loss of libido, memory impairment, ringing in the ears, rising cholesterol levels, swelling of the face, feet, or hands, and voice changes.

In contrast, excessive production of the thyroid hormones, which is much less common but not rare, is called Graves disease. Graves usually comes on slowly, starting with a feeling of general malaise, hair loss, hot flushes, increased sensitivity to such stimulants as coffee and bronchodilators, insomnia, periods of rapid heart beat or palpitations, and weight loss. Lab tests can confirm Graves disease, and the treatment choices range from wait and see (Graves can spontaneously resolve, though not often) to surgical removal of the thyroid gland, followed by lifelong medical replacement of the thyroid hormone. The problem with a chronically overactive metabolism, as in Graves, is that the accelerated heart rate and accelerated bone loss will cause premature cardiovascular disease and osteoporosis.

Sufficient iodine intake is critical for optimal thyroid function, and a lack can lead to a goiter, a lump on the thyroid. A goiter is usually benign and not cancerous, but nevertheless is indicative of thyroid trouble and always warrants professional medical evaluation. The Midwest was once known as the goiter belt because people there lived a long way from the sea, and all foods naturally high in iodine are harvested from the sea. Since the early 1950s, however, the FDA has required that all commercially available table salt must contain iodine. Many people today restrict their salt (sodium chloride) intake, sometimes unnecessarily, which may be a factor in the rising rates of thyroid trouble. Environmental pollution is another culprit.

Doctors often check for thyroid problems by using a blood test for TSH (thyroid-stimulating hormone) levels because this takes less time than hitting the Achilles tendon, instructing the patient in taking their morning temperatures, and asking all the questions that would reveal low thyroid function. The TSH test is a fairly good screening tool, but it is incomplete and should be accompanied by the above procedures. The standard range for normal TSH levels is considered to be 0.5–5.5, though I prefer to see TSH in the range of

0.5–2.0. The thyroid gland has to start working harder than optimum in order to function properly when TSH levels climb higher than 2.0. A good thyroid exam should always include feeling for the size and consistency of the gland. The doctor may ask you to swallow while gently touching your throat near the thyroid tissue. Ultrasound or biopsies may be needed if the gland is enlarged, hardened, or lumpy.

As mentioned above, a woman with hot flashes may have plummeting estrogen levels, or have heavy bleeding from excess estrogen, but the origin of the problem may be the thyroid gland, not the ovaries. In fact, when women do show high-estrogen symptoms, as for example, heavier, more frequent periods, or increased breast tenderness and bloating, my treatment approach is often to enhance thyroid function. I start with the nutritional suggestion to avoid the goiter-forming foods (the Brassica family, which includes bok choy, broccoli, Brussels sprouts, cabbage, kale, rutabaga, and turnips, all suppressive to the thyroid especially when eaten raw). I also advise increasing high-iodine foods in the diet, such as crustaceans, fish, and sea vegetables. Look for powdered kelp at your local supermarket or health food store and sprinkle at least one-quarter teaspoon onto savory foods daily if your energy is low. Kelp is not just high in iodine; it is also high in many other important trace minerals. Your body digests and absorbs it more readily than a pill because it is a food, not a processed supplement.

EFFECTS OF THYROID HORMONE ON VARIOUS ORGAN SYSTEMS

ORGAN	THYROID EXCESS	THYROID DEFICIENCY
Blood vessels	Open: warmer skin	Constricted: hypertension
Bones	Bone loss	Bone thickening
Heart	Increased heart rate	Decreased heart rate
Intestines	Loose stools	Constipation
Nerves	Feeling jittery	Feeling sluggish
Skin	Warm, smooth, moist	Rough, dry

If you need thyroid medication, consider taking it not with food because food seems to interfere with the absorption of most thyroid medications. You may be able to lower your dose, and when it come to prescription medicine, less is definitely better when possible.

Case Study: Low Thyroid Function

Lucinda, a forty-seven-year-old overweight woman, with sporadic but heavy menstruation and increasingly intense mood swings, came to the office complaining mainly of hair loss ("big gobs of hair come out in the shower"), weight gain (twenty pounds in the past four years), and a sensation of "tingling and numbness" in her feet. She also described having very little energy: just barely enough to "get through my day."

On examination, I found that all her deep tendon reflexes were subdued, and her Achilles tendon reflex was absent. Her skin was dry and slightly scaly, and her heart rate was regular but slow, with a pulse of 56. She said she exercised very little lately because of her general fatigue. These classic symptoms of low-thyroid function were borne out by basic lab work. I chose to begin Lucinda's therapy with a low dose of Armour thyroid, which is derived from the thyroid glands of sheep or pigs and provides a mix of T3 and T4, the two major thyroid hormones, in approximately the ratio found in humans.

Within three days, Lucinda reported that her energy was "much improved." After ten days on the Armour thyroid, she called the office to say that her hair had stopped falling out and she didn't need to use huge amounts of lotion on her hands, face, and legs anymore because her skin was not as dry as it had been. She added to these successes over the next six months by losing twenty-five pounds, thanks in part to having enough energy to resume her previous level of regular moderate exercise.

PART FOUR

How to Stay Healthy for a Long Time

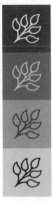

20.

Immune-System Basics

We hear a lot about the immune system these days. We hear about autoimmune diseases (lupus and multiple sclerosis, for example), about immunodeficiency diseases (HIV/AIDS), about immunizations (the flu shot and others), and about how stress and environmental pollution make our immune systems work harder than ever. What is the common thread between all these topics? What do medical scientists mean when they talk about the immune system? They are talking about your white blood cells. Inside the long leg and arm bones and the hip and rib bones is a fantastic substance called bone marrow, which is where new blood cells are created. All the blood cells—the red cells, the platelets, and the white cells—are created in the marrow. Platelets have no nucleus and are mostly used to help form scabs over a wound. Red blood cells transport oxygen and carbon dioxide. For now, I'm going to stick to a discussion of the colorless white blood cells.

White Blood Cells

There are many different types of white blood cells, all of which have different roles in keeping the body healthy. For example, there are the B cells, which are able to recognize foreign particles (antigens) in the bloodstream and immediately secrete an antibody to prevent the foreign particle from disrupting bodily functions. Antigens include bacteria and viruses, funguses, undigested food, pollutants such as solvents or noxious gases, synthetic chemicals, and even prions, the agents of Mad Cow disease and other strange brain diseases. When functioning properly, the body is extremely adept at differentiating between what is "self" and what is "not-self." Anything that is "not-self" most definitely does not belong in the bloodstream. The job of the B cells is to detect antigens (foreign particles) in the blood right away, and then create and secrete an antibody substance that mimics the antigen, effectively binding to it and blocking it from entering or attaching to body cells, where it can do damage. The B cells are definitely amazing, but the T cells, other lines of white blood cells, are even more sophisticated.

T cells

The T in T cells stands for thymus. You may not have heard of the thymus gland, but it is considered the master gland of the immune system. This gland is located approximately over the heart, and is about as large as a child's hand when you are young, but shrinks to the size of a flat walnut by late adulthood. The thymus gland can be thought of as a finishing school for basic white blood cells, which are educated by passing through the thymus gland and graduating as T cells. There are different types of T cells: helper T cells, killer T cells, suppressor T cells, and so on. These are the cells that destroy the antigens tagged by the B cells. The T cells are mostly involved in gobbling up (like a Pac-Man game) the antigen-antibody complex and shunting it into one or another of the organs of elimination where it can be flushed out of the body.

Lymph Nodes and Channels

Alongside the nerves and blood vessels throughout our entire body there exists another set of channels for drainage, the lymphatic channels, which are punctuated by nodes. These lymphatic channels can be thought of as the body's garbage collection system. Infections, and even newly formed cancerous tumors, are aggressively pushed into these drainage channels by the immune system. Although lymph nodes exist all over the body, they are closest to the surface in the armpits, the groin, behind the knees, and under the jaw. Because enlarged lymph nodes would indicate a deeper infection or a more serious problem, doctors almost always check for them as part of a physical exam.

Lymphatic drainage works through the contraction and relaxation of muscles. Unlike the blood vessels, there is no pump behind the lymphatic system. This is one reason why regular moderate exercise is so critical to good health—movement allows the body to efficiently transfer waste material into the channels of elimination, including the lymphatic channels, which ultimately drain into the kidneys. As you move, the muscles rhythmically contract, gently squeezing the channels of the lymphatic system. Another method for stimulating lymphatic circulation is to apply alternating hot and cold water to the skin, especially under the armpits, at the groin, and on the midback near the kidneys. I recommend that you chase every single hot shower with a good sixty seconds of pure cold water. A temperature differential of sixty degrees is required for a tonic effect. Hot expands the vessels; cold contracts them, flushing out toxins.

You can also dramatically reduce the healing time for a swollen joint, for example on a sprained ankle, by helping to pump out excess fluid with alternating hot and cold application, after you have used that famous first-aid technique RICE (rest, ice, compression, and elevation) for the first twenty-four to forty-eight hours. After the first forty-eight hours the alternating hot and cold immersion becomes much more effective for healing. First, immerse the foot (in the case of a sprained ankle) to above the ankle in warm to hot water for thirty seconds, and then plunge it into another container of ice cold water for ten seconds. Repeat this three times, twice daily, and always end with the cold immersion. In general, the use of this contrasting water therapy on your whole skin, every day, will greatly improve your capacity for eliminating toxins and will keep your skin toned. This leads us to that incredibly important organ of the immune system.

The Skin

The skin is the largest organ in the body. Skin is waterproof and full of oil glands that keep it lubricated and help make it resistant to water. The skin acts as a barrier for the protection and survival of our insides. The hostile world outside our bodies is replete with burning ultraviolet radiation, harsh winds, temperature swings, and bugs of all sorts. Our skin protects us from these insults, and keeps us warm in cold climates with the fat layer and cool in hot climates with sweat glands. Skin is covered all over with fine hair, which sends signals about the exterior environment to the brain through nerve impulses. Of all the senses, touch is perhaps the most critical to survival. It is now conventional wisdom that premature infants do much better if they are regularly touched while in incubation, even if they cannot see, smell, or hear. The outer layer of the skin sheds continuously and is completely replaced every month. You can help preserve the beauty and health of your skin by daily dry-skin brushing, a delightful and invigorating morning habit. (See Skin Brushing in Chapter 10.)

Diet and the Immune System

It is important to understand that bone marrow will generate only so many white blood cells. At some point, the ability of the immune system to keep up with the need for constant self-defense breaks down. Our immune system needs help to keep functioning for our lifetime benefit, which is where diet comes in. The food we eat is the most important contact between the outer environment and our delicate inner environment, because input is so constant. Think about it. We are basically a complicated tube covered by skin, with a hole at the top where food goes in, and a hole at the bottom where waste comes out. In and out, on a daily basis. If we're smart and our food choices are 100 percent nourishing, our food does not tax our immune system. Realistically, though, whether through gluttony, ignorance, poverty, or self-indulgence, ideal food choices are inconsistent. Even those of us who know what constitutes an excellent diet (lean clean protein, organic produce, plenty of pure water) will succumb to marketing strategies appealing to our palate instead of our intelligence. The problem with regularly eating foods that your body cannot properly digest is that now your immune system has to deal with that food.

Almost everyone is aware of food allergies, which can produce profound, life threatening, highly visible allergic reactions in some people. These reactions are rare, though, and usually involves peanuts, shellfish, or MSG (monosodium glutamate, often used as a flavor enhancer in Asian cuisine). More commonly, many people have food *sensitivities* they may not even be aware of. This means their bodies cannot optimally use food they are sensitive to for nutrition, nor readily break it down for elimination. These foods will cause some degree of intestinal irritation, requiring B cells to produce antigens and T cells to clear them from the body.

Foods That Cause Sensitivities

The most common food sensitivity offenders are wheat and dairy products. Wheat? The staff of life? Yes, it is true: many thousands of Americans are profoundly affected by wheat consumption. For some, eating wheat and other gluten-containing grains can be life threatening because of a condition called celiac disease, which is increasing in the United States. For many others the regular consumption of wheat-containing products will result in a variety of problems, including a bloated feeling, burning urination, carbohydrate cravings, fatigue, headaches, increased nighttime urination, irregular bowel function, irritability, joint pain, a painful tongue, a runny, stuffy nose, or even paranoid hallucinations.

In my clinical experience, the second most common food allergens are dairy products, including butter, ice cream, yogurt, and especially milk and cheese of all sorts. Goat's milk products may be a good substitute for those who find that cow's milk causes chest congestion, diarrhea, ear infections, malodorous flatulence, a stuffy or runny nose, vague abdominal pain, or even adult onset diabetes. Milk products are very common allergens and should be the first consideration for elimination in conditions characterized by excess mucus production. Most of the world's population does not consume dairy products after age two.

Other top food allergens are sugar, corn, soy, orange juice, nuts, tomatoes, and rarely, garlic, chocolate, and shellfish.

How to Determine Food Sensitivities

Usually, it will take several hours, or even days, after eating the offending food for an adverse reaction to appear. Symptoms of food sensitivities are variable, but can include changes in bowel habits, increased abdominal bloating and discomfort, increased mucus production (coughing up phlegm, stuffy nose), itchy ear/eyes/skin, and swelling, especially around the extremities. It can be difficult to sort out what is causing what since we eat many different foods daily. There are blood tests available which can quantify exactly how much the various foods tested are engaging the immune system, causing our B cells to secrete antibodies. (The blood tests usually look at ninety-six common foods.) The tests that scratch the skin to determine food sensitivities are useless; analyzing the blood is much more informative. I used food-allergy tests in my practice in the past, but I've discovered a much more economical, and often more accurate, method—the blood-type system.

Eat Right for Your Type

Despite all the hype, the work of Drs. James and Peter D'Adamo (father and son) has offered much real insight into determining which foods are wrong for any given individual. The basic idea is that a person's blood type, which is set for life and never changes, is expressed in every cell of the body. In other words, any cell (not just a blood cell) on your body could be used to determine whether you were one of the four major blood types: O, A, B, or AB. Because blood types are expressed through various proteins and carbohydrates protruding from the surface of our cells, it follows that different food proteins and carbohydrates will interact either favorably or disruptively with the cells that comprise the human body. The blood-type system guides us to eat foods that will not disrupt our cellular function, because disrupted cellular function ultimately results in accelerated aging and diminished immune competence. A very rudimentary overview of the system follows:

- **Blood type O** needs a high protein diet with no refined grains and plenty of fruits and vegetables. Wheat should be avoided altogether.

- **Blood type A** can eat eggs, fish, and fowl, but should avoid dairy products and red meat. Blood type A does well as a vegetarian. Some A types need to avoid nightshade foods (eggplant, peppers, potato, tomato), but this type can enjoy a diet higher in complex carbohydrates.

- **Blood type B** is the only type suited to dairy foods, but must avoid chicken (although chicken eggs are OK) and corn in all forms. B types generally don't do well with soy products, and should consume nuts sparingly.

- **Blood type AB**, a rare hybrid of A and B, can tolerate dairy better than A types but should mostly stick to fish and soy protein, plus, as with all the types, eat plenty of fruits and vegetables.

Vegetables (except tomatoes) are the least likely foods to cause health problems. Fruits are also well tolerated although some people get itchy, swollen throats from various fruits in the rose family, such as apples, some berries, and pears. *Eat Right for Your Type* and several subsequent books by Dr. Peter D'Adamo will give you all the information you need on this helpful system.

21.

Heart Disease

Half of all Americans who die before they are sixty-five die from heart disease. No question about it—heart disease is the leading cause of death in our country. Genetics is only part of your risk profile, so you need to learn about how to prevent premature cardiovascular disease even if it doesn't run in your family. There are several other important risk factors for early cardiovascular disease, including being overweight, smoking, and having high blood pressure, high cholesterol levels, or high homocysteine levels. All these risks are easy to determine.

Men Have More Heart Disease—True or False?

Men used to die of heart attacks, strokes, or congestive heart failure more frequently and younger than women, but the gap is closing. This is probably because today women smoke almost as much as men do, their lives are equally if not more stressful, and to earn the same amount of money as men, women have to work harder, even at the peaks of their careers.

Only a generation ago, there was very little heart-disease research conducted on women. All the standard drug models (such as beta-blockers, diuretics, and ACE-inhibitors) were developed based on studies conducted exclusively on men. Women were not considered candidates for early heart disease unless they had blatant symptoms, until recently. But women's cardiovascular function, although not radically different, is different enough from men's to warrant different diagnostic and treatment approaches. The blatant symptoms that were defined based on men were not blatant symptoms for women, and existing heart problems in women were likely to go undetected. For example, men are more susceptible to atherosclerosis, the buildup of plaque inside the blood vessels that puts more pressure on the heart and eventually causes heart attacks. Women are less prone to plaque buildup, but are much more likely than men to suffer from heart or blood-vessel spasms, which can lead to a heart attack or a stroke (similar to a heart attack, but in the brain). The major purpose of the red blood cells is to carry oxygen throughout the body via the blood vessels. If a blood vessel is in spasm, the proper flow of blood is inhibited, reducing the flow of oxygen to the brain, heart, and all the other vital organs. Irreversible damage occurs if the brain is deprived of a steady flow of oxygen for more than a few minutes. Even though an excess of oxygen is also damaging and causes tissue degeneration similar to rust (as discussed in Chapter 12), the right amount of oxygen is a paramount requirement for survival.

Heart Checkups

When you go to the doctor for a checkup, she/he will certainly pay attention to your heart. Your blood pressure is taken, the pulse is felt in several locations, and all four heart valves are listened to with the stethoscope. If the doctor suspects heart problems he/she may further examine your abdomen, chest, legs, and neck for more evidence. Sometimes x-rays or a treadmill stress test are recommended. The doctor may want to take your blood pressure in different positions, for example lying down, and then standing up. This will provide information about how quickly your vessels adjust to postural changes, which actually measures adrenal function. (Adrenaline keeps the blood pressure steady, whether you are lying down, upside down, or running.) The doctor will also want to know about your family history, your diet and exercise habits, and may also inquire about your social life, because being unhappy is bad for the heart. Some form of counseling may prove to be the best medicine for a sick heart. It is no coincidence that heart attacks occur most frequently on Monday mornings. If you chronically dislike your job, or your spouse, or the weather where you live, your heart will not be well.

Blood Pressure

Controlling blood-pressure is important for prolonged heart health. The pressure of the blood as it circulates around the body is an indirect evaluation of the function of the heart itself. Blood pressure is *not* the same as the pulse rate, which is the rate at which the heart is beating. Blood pressure is like air pressure in a bicycle tire; it's how hard the blood is pushing against the vessels that contain it. Blood pressure consists of two numbers. The upper number, the systolic, is a measure of this pressure at the extremities of your body. The lower number, the diastolic, is an indicator of the strength of the heart as a pump. A desirable reading is about 115/75, which is read "one-fifteen over seventy-five." Slightly lower is even better. There should be about a forty-point difference between the two numbers. Top athletes may have very low pulses, but their blood pressure should not be lower than 90/50. A reading of 140/90 is considered borderline hypertension, which means a problem is starting to develop. Blood pressure in the 200/150 range or above is a medical emergency. High blood pressure is destructive because many of the tissues of your body, such as the backs of the eyes, and the ultra-fine filtration devices in the kidneys, are extremely delicate and cannot sustain constant battering from fluid under high pressure. It would be like spraying a fire engine hose at your rose bushes for hours on end. High blood pressure can also be connected to kidney disease, which a doctor can help you figure out.

Cholesterol and CoQ$_{10}$

Blood cholesterol level testing is recommended for all adults at least once every five years. This test measures the levels of total cholesterol, HDL cholesterol (high-density lipoprotein—the "good" kind), LDL cholesterol (low-density lipoprotein—the "bad" kind), and the triglycerides in the blood serum. Many doctors simply look at the total blood cholesterol level, considering levels no higher than 200 to be acceptable (below 180 is considered optimal, 200–219 borderline high). However, this single number does not give the complete picture for each individual.

Sometimes blood pressure is high because cholesterol is clogging the arteries, a condition that, as mentioned previously, is more common in men. Women will often experience a mild rise in cholesterol levels as they go through menopause, without any accompanying rise in blood pressure. This is normal: as hormones wane, the liver wants to produce more hormone precursor, namely cholesterol. I strongly urge women to avoid cholesterol-lowering drugs if the ratio between their good (HDL) cholesterol and their total cholesterol is three or less. For example, if your total cholesterol is 240, some doctors might try to sell you statin drugs. However, if your HDL cholesterol (which removes cholesterol from the blood vessels and carries it back to the liver for recycling) is 80, then your ratio is three to one (240 divided by 80 equals 3). This is excellent! If your total cholesterol is 240 and your HDL is 40, however, your ratio is six to one, and that's not so good. In fact, treatment is required in this case, but not necessarily drugs. Several of my favorite natural cholesterol-lowering methods include garlic, niacin (vitamin B_3), Policosanol (derived from bee's wax), and red yeast rice (a rice found in Japan, taken in capsule form). I also like to use the plant medicine hawthorne (*Crataegus oxycantha*) for heart problems, because it not only lowers cholesterol by helping to digest fat, but also repairs the inner lining of the blood vessels, making them less prone to spasms and less likely to collect plaque.

Be aware that statins reduce levels of a critical cellular oxygenator, coenzyme Q_{10}. I always recommend a high dose of CoQ_{10}, 100 mg daily, to my heart patients, and I insist on it if they insist on taking statin drugs. Because CoQ_{10} helps convert water to oxygen inside the cells, it increases oxygen levels to an optimal threshold all over the body and reduces the burden on the heart of pumping oxygenated blood. I personally like to take a lower dose of CoQ_{10} before running, because it ensures a continuous flow of oxygen into the muscles, including the heart muscle and prevents the cramps caused by going into anaerobic respiration. Anaerobic respiration occurs, usually within twenty minutes of vigorous exercise, when the reserve of oxygen in the blood is depleted and the body has to use a different process to draw oxygen from the red blood cells into the muscle tissues. Unlike the carbon dioxide byproduct of aerobic respiration, the byproduct of anaerobic respiration is lactic acid, which causes tissue burn and achiness after exercise.

Plaque

Plaque is an aggregation of bacteria, calcium, and cholesterol in the inner lining of the blood vessels. Elevated cholesterol doesn't immediately make plaque buildup inevitable, though. To build up, plaque needs a roughened surface to grab onto, and then it slowly accumulates layer upon layer, just as it does on teeth. A diet high in colorful fruits and vegetables is the best remedy for healing the inner lining of blood vessels so they stay smooth and whole and offer no foothold for plaque.

Smoking

If you still smoke—stop! Be aware of all the ways cigarettes hook you, and find healthier substitutes. Substitute green tea and exercise if you use cigarettes for stimulants. Prunes and exercise are healthy laxatives. (Some smokers find that the nicotine in cigarettes can help stimulate a bowel movement, so quitting may cause temporary constipation.) If cigarettes are your stress controllers, use chamomile or licorice tea, deep breathing, exercise, meditation, walks outside, or yoga instead. If they substitute for companionship, call a friend, pay more attention to your family members, read a novel. Everyone knows that cigarette smoking causes lung cancer, and believe me, lung cancer is not a nice way to die. Surgery, chemotherapy, and radiation don't usually work, and you slowly asphyxiate, gasping for your final breaths.

Besides ruining the lungs, nicotine is also toxic to the heart and the cervix. I don't normally require annual Pap smears on women who are in mutually monogamous relationships and have a history of normal Paps (a Pap smear is a screening test for cervical cancer.) However, if my patient uses hormones or smokes, I do require an annual cervical sampling.

Quit, even if it's hard to do. Remember you *can* take a break—and live—without having a cigarette. Don't be fooled by movie or TV actors smoking; it is definitely not cool anymore.

Homocysteine

High homocysteine levels are independent markers of premature cardiovascular death, and are now considered to be more highly correlated with heart problems than high cholesterol. Don't be surprised if you have never heard of this because some doctors haven't either, although it has been widely discussed in the medical literature for the last eight years. Homocysteine is a byproduct of an amino acid found in meat, onions, cabbage, and a host of other foods, although that doesn't mean these foods are bad to eat. If a blood test determines that homocysteine levels in your blood are too high, it usually means you are deficient in certain B vitamins. Many doctors won't even test for homocysteine, because high levels are so easy and inexpensive to treat by taking B vitamins. However, some people can have high homocysteine levels despite good B-vitamin intake, so their problem is *absorption*, not inadequate ingestion, of the B vitamins.

In my family practice, I look at all the risk factors if someone is concerned about their heart health. If both parents died of heart disease and the person is overweight and has high cholesterol and high blood pressure, improving her/his weight will probably get both the cholesterol and the blood pressure into a more optimal range. Usually, I also monitor homocysteine levels and make sure my treatment brings them down to below nine. If, however, the only risk factor is slightly high cholesterol, and another doctor is pressuring them to take drugs, it is especially important to check homocysteine. If their homocysteine level is an optimal seven or less (fifteen is considered high in terms of cardiovascular risk), I'll reassure them about their heart. We'll continue to check the cholesterol/HDL ratio annually, because I am more interested in the ratio between total cholesterol and HDL cholesterol than just the total cholesterol. Don't get too hung up on the number 200. I will also advise the patient with slight to moderate total cholesterol elevation to use natural cholesterol-lowering methods such as improving their diet and increasing their exercise levels.

An increasingly common problem in the United States is celiac disease, a form of gluten intolerance in which gluten erodes the lining of the small intestine and inhibits nutrient absorption, in particular the absorption of the B vitamins. I check for celiac disease, which often shows up as loose stools and difficulty digesting grains, whenever I have a patient with good B-vitamin intake but higher than optimal homocysteine. Most high-gluten foods are grains, including barley, rye and spelt, with the biggest offender being wheat.

Weight Control

Blood pressure is often high when a person is overweight. If your blood pressure is high and you are carrying excess weight it is much more sensible to lose weight than to become dependent on prescription drugs. I have single-handedly discovered a foolproof, miraculous, no-calculator-needed method for achieving permanent weight loss. Here it is, the long-awaited nemesis of all diet plans: Burn More Calories Than You Eat.

Joking aside, there really isn't any other way to lose weight. The bottom line is always going to be to use up the calories faster than you consume them, by getting buff in the gym, housecleaning, running after kids, thinking, whatever. You need to burn about 500 calories to lose one pound of extra body weight. Water weight comes off easily and doesn't really count because what you want is less fat, not less water in your body. And fat isn't necessarily the worst thing to eat either, because a little goes a long way in terms of making you feel satisfied. Don't be fooled by the low-fat foods because they're loaded with refined carbohydrates. Read the labels. A small scoop of full-fat ice cream has about the same number of calories as a slightly larger scoop of low-fat ice cream, but you don't feel nearly as full after the low-fat variety. So you probably eat a little more, which puts you at an equal number of calories and gives you less taste. Besides, the extra sugar you get in the low-fat products turns to fat soon enough, unless it is immediately burned off with vigorous activity.

Diet Plan

Keep your diet plan simple. Balance the protein (about 20 to 40 percent) with the fat (about 15 to 30 percent) and the carbohydrates (30 to 65 percent) during any given day and at each meal. Look at your plate: There should be approximately equal amounts of protein (beans/eggs/fish/meat) and carbohydrates (grains/vegetables) evident, with a dollop of fat (dairy/nuts/oil). You should completely avoid processed food, especially burgers, fries, milk shakes, and sodas, and just about anything sold in fast-food stores. Choose whole foods, something that actually grew in the ground recently. A whole food is complete by itself, like an apple or a carrot. It's fine to mix ingredients and spice things up, but choose high-quality ingredients.

Making good food takes time, and a healthy diet plan is really more about time than calories. You must be committed to good health and not just settle for convenience. People want pills, sugar, and stimulants, and want them right this instant, so unfortunately they are widely available, to the detriment of our nation's health. Your health, and the health of your children and all of us, depends on stepping back and taking time to prepare meals with whole foods, to exercise regularly, and to sleep eight hours a night.

Reduce Salt, Increase Potassium

The World Health Organization recommends eating less than 5 grams of sodium (table salt is sodium chloride) daily. For those with heart problems, especially high blood pressure, 1 gram of sodium daily is optimal. Two small pieces of fried chicken from any fast-food establishment will contain about 3 grams of salt. A quarter-pound burger contains 1.5 grams of salt. Salt contributes to swelling because it retains fluid in the tissues outside the cells. Sugar does the same, though not as dramatically, but it will also lower your good cholesterol.

A critical mineral for healthy hearts is potassium, the counterpart to sodium in keeping fluids pumping in and out of the cells. Foods high in potassium include bananas and potatoes. If you have heart problems and do not regularly consume these foods, consider supplementing with 100 mg of potassium daily, but avoid oversupplementing.

What a Healthy Meal Looks Like
- ⅓ **Protein** (or more): beans (many different types), cheese (low-fat organic), eggs (cage free), fish (preferably not farmed), meat (free range if possible).

- **⅓ to ½ Carbohydrates** (or more): whole grains, such as barley, millet, oats, quinoa, rice, which all cook with 2 parts water to 1 part grain. Try to feature the colorful carbohydrates at least twice daily: beets, broccoli, carrots, chard, kale, peppers, spinach, squashes, sweet potatoes, or yams. Choose fresh and organic whenever possible. Eat lots of garlic and onions for heart health.

- **⅓ Fat** (or less): dairy products (organic), nuts/nut butters (keep these refrigerated so they don't go rancid), oil (coconut, flax, or olive). As stated in Chapter 16, although coconut oil is a saturated fat, it is a reasonable choice for stir-frying when used sparingly because it is more stable at higher heats than most fats, it is not hydrogenated, and it has no trans-fatty acids. It consists of 50 percent lauric acid, a good fat, and structurally is a medium chain triglyceride, which the body can metabolize efficiently and convert into energy rather than store as fat. Avoid anything fried or made with saturated or hydrogenated fat because they deteriorate your health rapidly.

The Perfect Snack

Fruit is the perfect snack! Fruit should be eaten by itself, apart from other food, because it digests rapidly and will ferment in the digestive tract if eaten at the same time as more slowly digested foods. Appreciate fruit as an amazing natural phenomenon each time you eat it. It's delicious, nutritious, and any remainders are biodegradable. Take your pick between crisp juicy apples, creamy bananas high in minerals, tasty berries to repair your blood vessels and restore eyesight, dates for an extra-sweet treat, succulent grapes, delectable mangoes, or scores of other tasty choices. What could be better?

Latest Scientific Guidelines on Food and Exercise

In September 2002, the Institute of Medicine (the medical branch of the National Academy of Sciences, and a major governmental advisor on health policy) released new guidelines on food and exercise. The new guidelines allow greater choice in the percentage of macronutrients (carbohydrates, fat, and protein) in the daily diet, but emphasize two important points.

1. The type of fat in the diet is very important. Avoid saturated fats (those that are solid at room temperature), especially hydrogenated fats such as margarine. These fats raise the levels of bad cholesterol (LDL) and increase the risk for cardiovascular disease.

2. Women over fifty are strongly urged to consume 21 grams of fiber daily. Younger women should get 25 grams daily. Food sources of fiber include apples, cereal products, legumes, onions, celery, sweet potatoes, and whole grains. While fiber itself has no nutritive value, it is crucial because it helps waste products move through the intestines, promoting healthy bowel movements. Fiber also inhibits fat and cholesterol absorption, stabilizes the blood-sugar balance, and slows digestion, which curbs hunger and allows for proper nutrient absorption.

The IOM made it very clear that any advice about diet must go hand in hand with advice about activity level. To quote one of the scientists, "We can't give recommendations on how much to eat unless we also comment on how much to burn." The bottom line, concluded the panel, is that Americans should get at least sixty minutes a day of moderately intense exercise, such as walking at pace of four miles per hour, calisthenics, golf without a cart, slow swimming, or leisurely bicycling. They added that these activities must be over and above housework and yard work.

Working Out

As you see from the table on page 152, leisurely walking, even daily, is no longer considered adequate exercise. According to the new recommendations, most Americans would be considered sedentary or as having a low active lifestyle. There is a direct relationship between heart disease, obesity, and lack of exercise. These factors are also linked, by the way, in a direct relationship to time spent viewing television. To get fit, we need to turn off the tube and work up to one hour daily of aerobic exercise, plus two sessions weekly of weight training. I add one to two stretching sessions to this formula.

Unless you have a physically demanding job, exercise rarely happens spontaneously and for most, it must be scheduled. I recommend workouts in the morning. If you have school-age children the kids are likely to be in school then, so you won't run out of time, a common excuse for not exercising. Try multi-tasking (normal for women). You can do professional reading while on an exercise bike. You can have brisk walking meetings with business colleagues. If you insist on watching TV, run on the treadmill, or lift some weights at the same time. You must honor your appointment to exercise, just as you honor your doctor or dentist appointments. It helps to hook up with an exercise buddy because you will be committed to that person also.

DAILY CALORIE REQUIREMENTS BASED ON HEIGHT/WEIGHT/ACTIVITY LEVEL*			
HEIGHT	**WEIGHT (LBS)**	**ACTIVITY LEVEL**	**CALORIES/DAY**
5'1"	98–132	Sedentary	1,548–1,694
		Low active	1,733–1,897
		Active	1,964–2,150
		High active	2,242–2,453
5'5"	111–150	Sedentary	1,676–1,842
		Low active	1,876–2,062
		Active	2,127–2,337
		High active	2,427–2,667
5'9"	125–169	Sedentary	1,808–1,994
		Low active	2,024–2,232
		Active	2,294–2,530
		High active	2,618–2,888

Low active = Walking thirty minutes a day at four miles per hour, or swimming thirty minutes a day.

Active = Walking thirty minutes a day at four miles per hour, plus thirty minutes of aerobics or cycling moderately per day.

High active = Walking for forty minutes a day at five miles per hour, plus forty minutes of doubles tennis, plus thirty minutes of cycling moderately per day.

*Chart courtesy of Dietary Reference Intakes for Energy, National Academies Press, 2002, reprinted in *Harvard Women's Health Watch* newsletter, November 2002).

Stay Positive

Be patient and stay positive about your changes toward a healthier lifestyle. These changes won't come overnight; you might take two steps forward, one step back. Don't throw in the towel just because you blew off one exercise commitment (or had one cigarette, or whatever). Tomorrow is a new day to start fresh. The human body *wants* positive feelings, and they are one of the greatest benefits of exercise. Vigorous exercise releases wonderful internal chemicals called endorphins, which make you feel happy and satisfied. Feeling good and cultivating a positive attitude will go a long way toward keeping you committed to your exercise program. Staying optimistic lowers your risk of dying of heart disease and cancer. It is never too late to become an optimist. Look forward, that's where you can make positive changes. Let go of the past; it's done and gone.

Beat the Dropout Odds

At New Year's, many people decide to get healthier, stop smoking, start exercising, lose weight. That's fine, but staying off the cigarettes, keeping up the exercising, and keeping off the weight is the real challenge. Your success with the initial commitment hinges on the day-to-day choices you make for the rest of your life. Here is a guide to help you stay with your exercise program.

- **Week One:** Attempting too much, too soon can lead to sore muscles, fatigue and maybe injuries. Working with equipment lacking proper instructions can lead to frustration and injuries. But don't give up. Begin slowly, and always warm up. Work at your own level, and gradually increase the duration and level of challenge. It's natural to feel awkward at this point—everyone was once a beginner. If you can, work with a personal fitness trainer for a few sessions to develop an incremental program. Talk to friends or acquaintances that you know are involved in the activity you have chosen as they are likely to be very willing to share tips.

- **Weeks Two to Four:** Enthusiasm can wane when you don't instantly lose all the weight, or if the hard body you want doesn't quite show through yet. Remember, permanent weight loss happens slowly. Aim for one pound weekly, or a maximum of two pounds weekly if you are more than 100 pounds overweight. One pound weekly means fifty pounds a year. Stick with it. Keep in mind that internal changes occur before any benefits are externally visible. Consider adding a different activity to your routine (switch out one day of aerobics for a spinning class, or a trot around the track) to prevent boredom.

- **Weeks Twelve through Month Six:** By now you have noticed some physical changes. You've developed leaner muscle mass, improved your endurance and aerobic capacity, reduced your blood pressure, and maybe had some weight loss that shows. Undoubtedly, unforeseen variables will arise that tempt you to veer away from your exercise routine—illness, out-of-town visitors, vacation, and so on. Use your willpower to stay focused through this critical period and don't lose your gains. It is time to appraise your enjoyment level of your routine, because it is no longer productive to force yourself to perform an activity you don't enjoy. Maybe you need to find a group, or start to work out solo. Maybe you need to switch the time of day you exercise. Maybe you need to spend more time outside, or less, depending on the weather. It's OK to shake up the routine, but stay with it and focus on the benefits that have already accrued.

- **Months Six through Nine:** At this point, many people reach a plateau. You have probably gained lean muscle, improved your endurance and stamina, and lost weight. Your blood pressure and cholesterol are probably both down, and you look a lot better. But the thrill may not be there anymore. Don't be discouraged. Think of it this way—feeling good is now normal for you. You must think long-term and recognize that you may need new challenges or a greater variety in your workouts to stay motivated. Try a new sport, machine, or class. Compete in a local low-pressure race. Get a new pair of shoes or a new exercise outfit. If you make it through to the one-year mark of regular exercise, you are almost 100 percent guaranteed to be hooked for life.

Help your daughters and sons get into the exercise habit early. There is no question that using your fork and your running shoes judiciously will prevent most premature deaths from heart disease.

Weight Training

For those who prefer not to use the gym, a few sets of hand weights in your own home can provide all you need for strength-training exercise. Strength training with weights, also called resistance training, will enhance your balance, improve your appearance, increase your bone density, and slow the aging process overall. The following strength-training exercises are appropriate for all ages:

Ten Basic Strength Training Exercises

For healthy adults of all ages, groups such as the American College of Sports Medicine and the Centers for Disease Control recommend strength training two to three days a week, incorporating eight to ten exercises that involve major upper- and lower-body muscle groups. The following exercises will help train the muscles in your arms, shoulders, chest, abdomen, back, hips, and legs. Beginners should practice two to three times per week, starting with a weight load that allows a maximum of eight to twelve repetitions (ten to fifteen repetitions for women 50 and older) per exercise. When exercising one leg or arm at a time, do a set of repetitions on one side before changing to the other side.

SEATED, WITH HAND WEIGHTS

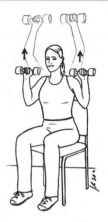

1. Overhead Press

Start with your upper arms close to your sides, elbows bent, and forearms perpendicular to the floor. Your palms should face forward and weights should be at shoulder level. Slowly press the weights upward until your arms are extended (don't lock your elbows). Weights should be slightly forward, not directly over your head. Pause. Slowly return to the starting position.

2. Forward Fly

Start by holding the weights about 12 inches in front of your chest with your elbows up and slightly bent (as if you're embracing a large beach ball). Lean forward at a slight angle, bending from your hips and keeping your back straight. Slowly try to make your shoulder blades touch behind you, letting the movement pull your elbows back as far as possible. Pause. Slowly return to the starting position.

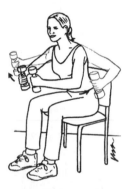

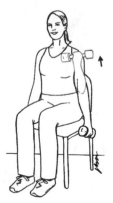

3. Biceps Curl

Hold a weight in each hand, arms extended straight down at your sides. Slowly raise the weight in one hand toward your shoulder, rotating your forearm as you lift so that the palm of your hand faces your shoulder. Do not move your elbow as you perform this movement. Pause. Slowly lower the weight to the starting position.

SEATED, WITH ANKLE WEIGHTS

4. Knee Extension

Sit with your knees 6 inches apart. Place a small rolled towel under the lower thigh of the leg you will work first. Slowly raise your foot, extending your leg until your knee is as straight as possible. Flex your foot, pointing your toes back toward you. Pause. Relax the foot. Lower it to the floor.

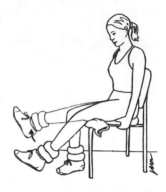

STANDING

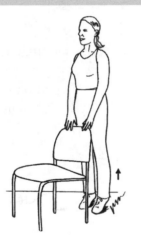

5. Plantar Flexion

Place your fingertips lightly on the back of a chair and stand tall. Slowly rise onto the balls of your feet; hold for 3 seconds, then slowly lower. If this is too easy, rise on one leg with the other bent at the knee.

6. Hip Extension

Wearing ankle weights, hold onto a chair back and slowly raise one leg straight out behind you. Lift the leg as high as possible without bending your knee or lowering your upper body forward more than 45 degrees. Pause. Slowly lower your leg.

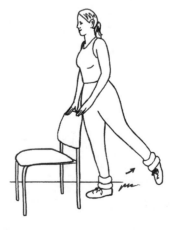

7. Hip Flexion

Wearing ankle weights, stand behind a chair, with your fingertips touching the chair back. Slowly bring one knee up toward your chest, without bending at your waist. Slowly lower your foot to the floor.

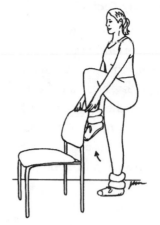

ON THE FLOOR

8. Side Leg Raise

Wearing ankle weights, lie on the floor on your right side. Bend your right leg slightly behind you. Your left leg should be straight, resting on top of the right knee. Support your head with your right hand; place your left hand on the floor in front of you for support. Slowly lift your left leg straight up, holding your torso still. Pause. Slowly lower your leg. After doing one or two sets of repetitions, repeat, lying on your left side.

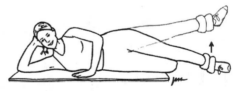

9. Chest Press

Lie on your back with your knees bent and your feet flat on the floor, hip distance apart. Extend your elbows out from your body and rest them on the floor. Hold the weights directly above your elbows. Slowly press upward until your elbows are straight. Pause. Slowly lower the weights.

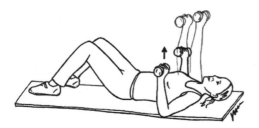

10. Tummy Tuck

Lie on your back with your
knees bent and your feet on
the floor, hip distance apart.
Slowly press the small of your
back into the floor, and tilt
your pelvis up toward your

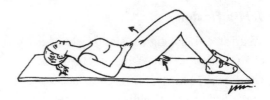

face. Your pelvis and lower buttocks will rise a few inches off the floor (place
your hand on your abdomen to feel your muscles working). Pause. Slowly
lower your pelvis.

Exercises courtesy of *Harvard Women's Health Watch* newsletter, August 2000.

22.

Reduce Your Risk of Cancer Now!

The "C" word strikes terror into our hearts. We all know someone who has suffered with cancer and most of us know people who have died from it. Many of us have already had cancer. It is epidemic. The war on cancer rages on because it is the second leading cause of premature death (after heart disease), and sophisticated new diagnostic and treatment strategies do not seem to be keeping pace with the increased incidences of cancer. Understanding something about why cancer is increasingly prevalent can help you formulate a plan for its prevention.

Basic Facts about Cancer

In a healthy person, cells divide, grow, and replace themselves in an orderly way, regulated by the nucleus (center) of each cell, where the genetic information is stored. When the genes that control normal cell functions fail for a variety of reasons, such as aging, improper nutrition, stress, or toxic burden, the cell becomes sick and starts dividing and multiplying out of control. A mass of these uncontrolled cells is called a tumor. Some of these tumors eventually stop growing, and these are considered benign (harmless). Malignant (cancerous) tumors, however, continue to grow and ultimately invade healthy tissues, use up the body's nutritional stores, and disrupt normal body functions.

There are more than two hundred different types of cancer, and more than 2 million people in the United States are diagnosed with a new case of cancer each year. Lung cancer is still the most deadly, and is mostly preventable by not smoking or being exposed to secondhand smoke. If you still smoke, get some help to quit now. Hormonal cancers of the breast, ovaries, and prostate are also quite prevalent. Brain and blood cancers are surprisingly common, particularly among children. About one million new cases of skin cancer are diagnosed yearly, and most could have been avoided with adequate protection against excess sun exposure. However, inadequate sun exposure, which leads to a vitamin D deficiency, is also a risk factor for many cancers, including breast cancer. So you do need some sun, but if you live south of the horizontal middle of the United States, avoid direct sunlight on unprotected skin between the hours of 10:00 A.M. and 2:00 P.M.

Seven Major Warning Signs of Cancer

1. Any persistent change in bowel habits or bladder function, such as seeing blood in your urine or stool, or being unable to pass urine or a stool, or experiencing pain from urination or passing a stool. These are possible markers for bladder or rectal cancers.

2. Any sore that does not heal anywhere on your body. If you have a patch of skin that stays chronically irritated, oozy, or abnormally itchy, check with a doctor. These are potential markers for skin cancers.

3. Unusual bleeding or discharge including abnormal vaginal bleeding or discharge, blood in the stool, or coughing up blood. Two weird periods per year are normal, however, because the menstrual cycle may just be disrupted from changes in your diet, stress, or travel. If your menses are very heavy, or persistently irregular, that doesn't mean it is a cancer of the female organs, but you should have it evaluated by a doctor.

4. A thickening or lump in the breast or elsewhere. A tumor is tissue growth that is out of control. Normal tissue will grow until the wound is filled in or the skin damage has been repaired. Cancerous growth is not normal and doesn't stop, but just keeps on growing. Lumps and bumps don't always mean cancer, but they should be evaluated right away, especially if they are actively growing.

5. Persistent indigestion or difficulty swallowing. Eating, swallowing, digestion, and bowel movements are not supposed to be painful or difficult. Digestive difficulties may signal cancerous tumors or ulcers along the digestive tract and should be checked right away.

6. Recent change in the size or color of a wart or mole. The ABCDs of figuring out if one of these skin growths is problematic are: A = area, B = border, C = color, and D = depth. If the Area of the skin growth is enlarging,

especially if it is growing rapidly, that's a bad sign. Other bad signs are when the Borders of the skin growth are ragged or irregular looking, and if the Color of the mole or wart is mixed—that is, part light brown, part black, part pink, part bluish. Finally, if the Depth of the skin growth is more than two millimeters, it should be biopsied to rule out cancer. Sometimes a mole is large and protrudes quite a bit but it is not cancerous. Nevertheless, your doctor may recommend its removal, particularly if it's somewhere on your body where it gets rubbed or irritated a lot (such as the midback, at the bra clasp, or around the waistline).

7. A nagging, hacking cough or hoarseness that last more than several weeks. These are possible markers for lung or throat cancer. There could also be a primary tumor in the breast, which could metastasize to the lungs before the breast tumor is caught.

Cancer Risk Factors

Genetics plays a small role in the likelihood of acquiring cancer; the bulk of the risk lies in environmental exposures. Most cancers today would be greatly reduced if our environment (air, water, consumer and medical products, the workplace) was not so contaminated. The average American is increasingly exposed to harmful chemicals, industrial carcinogens, and solvents present in cleaning solutions, cosmetics, pesticides, plastics, and processed food. Two documented but little-known risk factors for ovarian cancer are dyeing your hair regularly and using prescription antidepressant medication. Breast-cancer risks include being overweight, being exposed to environmental pollution, using prescription hormones, and wearing ill-fitting bras. In October 2002, Marin County, California, received an unprecedented $1 million grant from the Centers for Disease Control (CDC) to study the role that pollution played in the 72-percent jump in breast cancers there during the 1990s. Although the results have not yet been published, it is important to note that the study was begun on the assumption that pollution is the culprit, and this assumption has federal money behind it. Brain, blood, and bone cancers can often be traced to electromagnetic frequencies, high doses of radiation, and exposure to toxins such as dioxin, a bleach. At least 35 percent of cancers are directly related to poor nutrition. Eating two to three whole fruits and two to three cups of freshly cooked or raw vegetables daily will greatly enhance your ability to withstand the increasing devastation caused by internal and external pollution.

Reducing Toxic Exposure

Reducing or phasing out toxins is possible within our lifetimes *if* we get involved at a grass-roots level. There are many ways you can contribute to making the planet less toxic. At a personal level, you can choose to minimize your use of plastics. Use canvas bags for your shopping. Keep them in the car or near the handbag you use when you go shopping. Neither paper nor plastic bags are the best choice at the checkout line. If you get in the habit of using cloth bags, your children and grandchildren will imitate you. Then, as consumer demand decreases, production of plastics will diminish. Recycle whatever you can. Look into your local resources. Buy merchandise on eBay or at local thrift stores. Take care of your car, computer, and fax machine and use them until the bitter end. Avoid buying personal-care products that contain harmful chemicals, and tampons and menstrual pads that use bleached material. I recommend using natural sea sponges, or washable organic cotton pads to collect menstrual blood. Another good option is the rubber Keeper Cup, which will last a lifetime. Read labels and ask yourself if you really need the product if you see long words with syllables such as butyl, cetyl, ethyl, or propyl. Avoid dumping toxic chemicals into your mouth (sodas), onto your head (many shampoos and conditioners) or into the water supply (dish/laundry detergents containing phosphates and other chemicals). Vote for political leaders who care about the environment. Those who don't are stupid and greedy, and there's no excuse for that anymore. Drastic reform is needed now. Together, we can make a difference.

"Mainstream industry consumer products—foods and beverages, cosmetics and toiletries, and household products, including home, lawn, and garden pesticides—contain a wide range of undisclosed carcinogens which pose major, but generally unrecognized, avoidable risks of cancer." This quote is from "Reversing the Cancer Epidemic," an essay by Samuel S. Epstein, M.D., a professor of occupational and environmental medicine at the University of Illinois Medical Center, medical director of the Cancer Prevention Coalition in Chicago, IL, author of ten books, and a consumer watchdog. Look for his online reports on dirty consumer products at www.preventcancer.com.

Readily Modified Risk Factors

Environmental pollution is the number-one risk factor for cancer, but this will slowly improve with your help. Until then, you can get more immediate results by controlling the two factors that are undeniably linked to health and longevity: your diet and your level of physical activity. Women who gain weight at menopause are more vulnerable to breast cancer, and those who don't exercise are more likely to acquire breast, colon, and stomach cancers. Get into the exercise habit now because it can greatly help you manage your menopause. Excessive alcohol intake is another risk factor for breast, colon, liver, pancreatic, and throat cancers. Women are advised to hold their consumption of alcoholic beverages down to two ounces daily. And don't save up for the weekend—binge drinking confers the highest risk.

If you already have cancer, keep exercising. Physical activity can improve the outcome for cancer patients. It helps relieve depression and anxiety, and helps you maintain an optimal weight. Even a short daily walk can make a difference.

Anti-Cancer Diet

The twelve top cancer-fighting foods are:

1. Beans (dried beans, lentils, split peas)

2. Carotenoid-rich fruits and vegetables that are deep green, orange, red, and yellow

3. Citrus fruits

4. Cruciferous vegetables (broccoli, cabbage, kale)

5. Fiber-rich foods (beans, fruits, vegetables, and whole grains)

6. Coldwater fish varieties such as salmon, trout, tuna

7. Garlic

8. Green tea

9. Medicinal varieties of mushrooms including maitake, reishi, and shiitake

10. Nuts and seeds

11. Soybeans (organic miso, soy nuts, tempeh, tofu)

12. Yogurt (organic)

Explore which of these healing foods works best for you and your family.

Tampering with our food supply is unlikely to promote good health. Breast milk, even from mothers exposed to pesticides, will always be better than infant formula. Whole grains are infinitely more nutritious (and delicious) than refined flour products, which have less fiber and lower vitamin, mineral, and natural oil contents. As my nutrition teacher said, try to only eat foods that would rot, but eat them before they do. Since women are often the ones involved with food preparation, we have a fantastic opportunity to improve our own health and that of our families, our communities, and ultimately the planet. I advise my patients to ask themselves eight basic questions when devising the most healthful diet for themselves and their families:

1. How did your ancestors eat? The more pure blood you have from a specific ethnic group, the more important it is to be guided by the traditional dietary habits of your clan.

2. Does your food display lots of natural colors? When you are preparing a meal, do you notice bright red, burgundy, deep green, natural yellow, orange, violet? Colors are good, but only if they are naturally occurring. Avoid artificially colored foods; food dyes are potent chemicals and are linked to brain disorders, including adult attention deficit disorder and seizures.

3. Are the ingredients of your meal whole foods? Use deepwater wild fish, fresh fruit, organic produce, range-fed animals, real sea salt, whole grains. Shop in the produce section, which is usually at the edge of the grocery store. Avoid processed foods, which are low in fiber and short on nutrients. They are extremely expensive relative to the nutritional value they deliver and will undermine your health.

4. Are you buying anything containing sugar? Make every effort to limit your sugar intake. Whole fruit is always a better choice than candy or a sugary baked food, because fruit is high in vitamin C and fiber. The worst sugar is corn syrup, which will make you fat and diabetic and promote heart disease. Avoid all artificial sweeteners, including aspartame, sucralose, and saccharin. Minimize consumption of dextrose, glucose, and sucrose.

5. Is your protein lean and clean? That means fish or wild game, and chicken or turkeys raised outside a cage and free of hormones and antibiotics. That also means cage-free eggs and organically grown legumes, nuts, and seeds.

Protein is the nutritional backbone of your immune cells, which can destroy cancer cells if they remain healthy.

6. Are your fat choices good fats? Can you recognize a bad fat? The good fats are liquid at room temperature and include borage, flax, olive, and evening primrose oils. Organic canola, safflower, and sunflower oils are OK, but avoid corn, peanut, and generic vegetable oils. Fish oils (high in omega-3s) are wonderful for your health. They protect your blood vessels, your eyes, your heart, and your skin. Except for butter and coconut butter, both eaten sparingly (see Chapter 16), the really bad fats are solid at room temperature. Never cook with lard, margarine, or Crisco.

7. Do you have a balanced ratio of carbohydrates, fat, and protein at each meal? The carbohydrates (grains, vegetables) should comprise a little more than one-third of the meal, the protein (beans, eggs, fish, meat) should be about one-third of the meal, and the fat (dairy products, salad dressing, cooking oil) should be less than one-third of the meal.

8. Are you spicing up your meals with natural flavors? Many kitchen herbs confer great health benefits. Garlic, for example, is a top-notch cancer-fighter. You can bake it whole or use it as a flavoring in sauces and salad dressings. Ginger is terrific for warding off the beginning of a cold and helps calm an upset stomach. Mint is cooling. Oregano, rosemary, sage, and thyme are antimicrobial (they can help kill disease-causing bacteria, fungi, and viruses). Licorice can heal stomach ulcers and reduce the stress response. Parsley is full of oxygenating chlorophyll and can treat bad breath. Turmeric is a powerful anticancer root, and gives a pleasant flavor and orange-gold color to broths or rice.

The bottom line with cancer prevention is to avoid chemicals, drink plenty of pure water, eat colorful foods, and exercise daily. Enjoy!

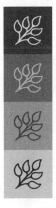

Conclusion

Going through menopause is inevitable. You are likely to experience changes in your body, mind, and spirit before, during, and after the cessation of menses. Because you are an individual, you'll have your own unique way of living through these changes, but ultimately you will become even more of the woman you are now. These changes are exciting, but will sometimes feel overwhelming. That's natural—they are big changes. You needn't suffer through them, however, and menopause should not be viewed as an incurable disease. Hot flashes, moodiness, and poor memory can all be treated naturally and effectively.

I invite you to believe in your complete wellness and to invest energy and time in your health. There is really no such thing as being too healthy, so go for it: Eat right. Sleep enough, every night. Enjoy the deepening of your relationships, including the important relationship to yourself. This book has introduced you to a variety of safe, effective methods for extending your life and health. Reach for those stars, through perimenopause, menopause, and forever!

Resources

Gen MacManiman
3023 362nd Avenue SE
Fall City, Washington 98024
1-425-222-5587
Castor oil in roll-on form.

**International Academy of
  Compounding Pharmacists**
P.O. Box 1365
Sugarland, Texas 77487
1-800-927-4227
www.iacprx.org
*These chemists formulate bioidentical
hormones.*

J.R. Carlson Laboratories
15 College Drive
Arlington Heights, Illinois
  60004-1985
1-888-234-5656
1-847-255-1600
www.carlsonlabs.com
Suppliers of high-quality supplements.

Mayway Corporation
1338 Mandela Parkway
Oakland, CA 94607
1-800-2MAYWAY
www.sales@mayway.com
*Distributes Plum Flower Company (Chinese
patent medicine company) and Seven
Treasures for Beautiful Hair, a patented
combination of several herbal remedies.*

PhytoPharmica
825 Challenger Drive
Green Bay, WI 54311
1-800-553-2370
www.phytopharmica.com
*Makers of Osteoprime Forte, a high-
quality bone-building supplement*

**Professional Compounding
  Centers of America**
9901 South Wilcrest
Houston, Texas 77099
1-800-331-2498
www.pccarx.com
*If there is no compounding pharmacist in
your area (check the yellow pages), you
can contact the organization above.*

Lexxus International
12901 Hutton drive
Dallas, TX 75234
1-972-241-6525
1-604-533-4425
www.lexxusinternational.com
Makers of Viacreme, a vaginal lubricant.

Traditional Medicinals
4515 Ross Road
Sebastopol, CA 95472
1-800-543-4372
1-707-823-8911
www.TraditionalMedicinals.com
Female Sage is one of their high-quality herbal tea products.

Visit www.naturopathic.org to find a licensed naturopathic physician in your area.

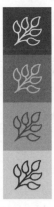

References

Ayres, Ed. "Rogue Corn on the Loose." *World Watch* Vol. 15:6. (November/ December 2002): 11–18.

Baur, Cathryn. *Acupressure for Women.* Freedom, CA: The Crossing Press, 1987.

Birdsall, Tim. "The Biological Effects and Clinical Uses of the Pineal Hormone Melatonin." *Alternative Medical Review* Vol. 1:2. (1996): 94–101.

Brinker, Francis J. *Formulas for Healthful Living.* Sandy, OR: Eclectic Medical Publications, 1995.

Cambridge Heart Antioxidant Study (acronym CHAOS) is an ongoing trial studying the effectiveness of vitamin E in preventing non-fatal heart attacks. The most recent discussion of this trial is discussed in Niki, E., and Noguchi ,N. "CHAOS (Cambridge Heart Antioxidant Study)." *Nippon Rinsho* Supplement 59:3 (March 2001): 448–451.

Carlson, John R. "Briefly," *News from John* newsletter. Arlington Heights, IL, 2002. www.carlsonlabs.com.

Chopra, Deepak. "Secrets of Much Better Sleep." *Bottom Line* (June 1997) Del Mar, CA.

D'Adamo, Peter J., and Catherine Whitney. *Eat Right for Your Type.* New York, NY: Putnam Publishing Group, 1996.

English, J. "A Natural Approach to Enhancing Sexual Libido and Performance," *Vitamin Research News* Vol. 16:9 (September 2002): 1–4.

Epstein, Samuel S. "Reversing the Cancer Epidemic." Tikkun, Vol. 17, No. 3, 56–65, May/June 2002. Online reports on dirty consumer products at www. preventcancer.com

Fleischmann, E.B. "Bio-Identical HRT." School paper, Bastyr University, Bothell, WA, 1998.

Ford, Gillian. *What's Wrong With My Hormones?* Newcastle, CA: Desmond Ford Publications, 1994.

Gaby, Alan R., and Jonathan Wright. "Nutrients and Bone Health," monograph. Baltimore, MD: Wright/Gaby Nutrition Institute, August, 1998.

Guyton, Arthur C., and John E. Hall, *Textbook of Medical Physiology.* 10th ed. Philadelphia, PA: WB Saunders Co., 2000.

Hudson, Tori S., Leanna Standish, et al. "Clinical and Endocrinological Effects of a Menopausal Botanical Formula." *Journal of Naturopathic Medicine* 7:1. (1998): 73–77.

Hudson, Tori S. "Perimenopause and Menopause." *The Townsend Letter for Doctors and Patients* (November 2002).

Birdsall, Tim. *Ipriflavone.* monograph, Sandpoint, ID: Thorne Research Inc, 1999.

Jubiz, William. *Endocrinology: Logical Approach for Clinicians.* New York, NY: McGraw-Hill, 1985.

Kane, Emily. "Getting to the Root of Hair Loss." *Let's Live Magazine* (August 1998), p. 56.

Katzen, Mollie. *The Moosewood Cookbook.* Berkeley, CA: Ten Speed Press, 1977.

Kolata, Gina. "Rush to Fill Void in Menopause Drug Market." *The New York Times,* (September 1, 2002), page 1, section C.

Laine, Kristen. "Hot Flash, Revised." *Delicious Living.* (September 2002): 62–68.

Lark, Susan. *The Lark Letter* newsletter, Potomac, MD: Phillips Health, LLC, September 2002, page 3.

Love, Susan. *Dr. Susan Love's Hormone Book.* New York, NY: Three Rivers Press, 1997.

Lu, N. "Conquering the HRT Dilemma with TCM," (conference handout) Vol 4:3. (Fall 2002): page 1. Traditional Chinese Medicine World Foundation, New York, NY.

Marchbanks, P.A., et al. "Oral contraceptives and the risk of breast cancer." *New England Journal of Medicine* Vol. 346 (June 27, 2002): 2025–2032.

Murray, Michael T., and Joseph E. Pizzorno. *Encyclopedia of Natural Medicine.* Rocklin, CA: Prima Publishing, 1995.

Murray, Michael. "Melatonin: miracle or hype?" *American Journal of Natural Medicine* Vol. 3:1. (January/February 1996): 5–7.

Niewoehner, Catherine B. *Endocrine Pathophysiology.* Madison, CT: Fence Creek Publications, 1998.

Ogletree, R.L., and R.G. Fischer. "The Top 10 Scientifically Proven Natural Products" booklet in *Natural Source Digest.* Brandon, MS, 1997.

Robb-Nicholson, C. "Why researchers stopped the Women's Health Initiative study of estrogen and progestin and what this means for you." *Harvard Women's Health Watch.* (September 2002): page 1.

Robbins, John. *Diet for a New America: How Your Food Choices Affect Your Health, Happiness and the Future of Life on Earth.* New York, NY: Bantam Press, 1987.

Robbins, John. *The Food Revolution: How Your Diet Can Help Save Your Life and Our World.* Berkeley, CA: Conari Press, 2001.

Schlosser, Eric. *Fast Food Nation: The Dark Side of the All-American Meal.* New York, NY: Houghton Mifflin, 2001.

"Taking Hormones and Women's Health: Choices, Risks and Benefits" booklet, Washington, DC: National Women's Health Network, 2000.

The Vitamin E Fact Book. LaGrange, IL: Vitamin E Research and Information Service (VERIS), 1990.

Wright, Jonathan V., and John Morgenthaler. *Natural Hormone Replacement: for Women Over 45.* Petaluma, CA: Smart Publications, 1997.

Index

About the Author

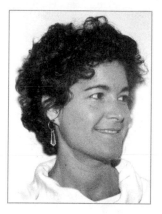

Emily A. Kane, N.D., L.Ac., graduated from Harvard University in 1978. After a decade working in performing arts, she graduated from Bastyr University with doctorate training in naturopathic medicine and master's level training in acupuncture and Eastern medicine in 1993. Dr. Kane is a former senior editor of the *Journal of Naturopathic Medicine*, the scientific, peer-reviewed journal of the American Association of Naturopathic Physicians, and now contributes frequently to *Let's Live* magazine. Visit www.DrEmilyKane.com for a library of published articles, contact information, and health retreat and workshop news. Dr. Kane resides in Juneau, Alaska, most of the year, where she teaches yoga and maintains a clinical practice. She winters in Hilo, Hawaii.